W9-BCQ-181

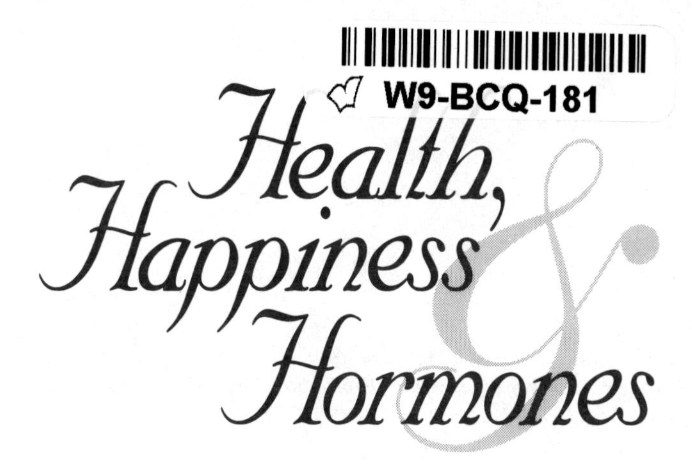

Health, Happiness & Hormones

One Woman's Journey Towards Health After a Hysterectomy

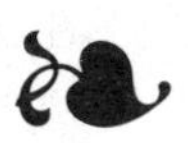

Arlene Swaney

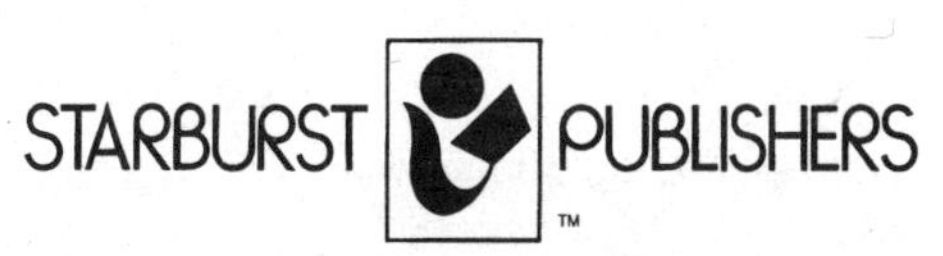

P.O. Box 4123, Lancaster, Pennsylvania 17604

To schedule Author appearances write:
Author Appearances, Starburst Promotions, P.O. Box 4123
Lancaster, Pennsylvania 17604 or call (717) 293-0939

The Publisher and its representatives take no responsibility for the validity of any material contained in this book. Neither shall the publisher be responsible for any possible consequence resulting from the use of material contained in this book. Nor does this book take the place of a physician's recommendations.

There are no warranties which extend beyond the educational nature of this book. Therefore, the publisher shall have neither liability nor responsibility to any person with respect to any loss or damage alleged to be caused, directly or indirectly, by the information contained in this book.

Credits:
Cover art by Terry Dugan Design

HEALTH, HAPPINESS & HORMONES

Copyright © 1996 by Starburst, Inc.
All rights reserved

This book may not be used or reproduced in any manner, in whole or in part, stored in a retrieval system or transmitted in any form by any means, electronic, mechanical, photocopy, recording, or otherwise, without written permission of the publisher, except as provided by USA copyright law.

First Printing, March, 1996

ISBN: 0-914984-72-1
Library of Congress Catalog Number 95-69734
Printed in the United States of America

To my *husband,*
who stood by me with love and patience
throughout the writing of this book,
and
to our *children* and their *families*—
especially our precious *grandchildren.*

Contents

1

The Hysterectomy

I had misgivings when, in 1980, my physician said he wanted me to have a complete hysterectomy. True, it would end inconvenient, heavy periods that seemed to come one right after another.

On the other hand, the thought of having my ovaries and uterus removed was scary. I worried still more when an older friend told me I'd be sorry, that I'd never feel the same again. Was it true or just one of those old wives' tales? I wondered.

I never questioned my doctor about estrogen replacement until a second friend, who'd also had a hysterectomy, said she regularly got estrogen shots. But when I asked my doctor about estrogen, he said it wasn't necessary.

I had never read anything about estrogen, but I did have faith in my doctor so I didn't question his reply. I figured, "He knows best."

The night before I entered the hospital, I couldn't sleep. I was flooded with apprehension and fear throughout the night. My anxiety increased just before I was wheeled into the operating room. But I'm usually cheerful, so I rationalized, "It's too late. I can't back out now. I'll just have to go ahead with this."

Moments later the anaesthetic took hold and the next thing I remember is my husband Bob at my side in the recovery room telling me that the operation went well.

Unlike my roommate who experienced post-hysterectomy problems, and six women who'd had the same operation just before me, I recovered quickly. Even my doctor expressed his delight when he released me from the hospital in less than a week.

While recuperating at home, I fretted about the hysterectomy and whether I'd made a wise decision. But ten days later when my doctor removed the stitches and announced I was free to do anything I felt up to, those misgivings disappeared.

"It's over," I thought. "Why not just be thankful that I don't have those awful periods to contend with anymore and get on with my life."

People always described me as a cheerful, positive person, the kind of person who could see the glass as half full rather than half empty.

My life revolved around my husband and three sons who were teenagers at the time. Church also was important. I was active in Bible study groups at Rogers Heights Christian Reformed Church and frequently went on church outings. And many of the friends we made through the years were just as active in church as we were.

But over the next seven years, my health deteriorated for no apparent reason. Visiting one doctor after another in hopes of finding out what was wrong and what I had to do to get better, I experienced so much emotional stress that I frequently thought about suicide. Fortunately, my faith in God sustained me.

"Never a weakness that He doth not feel
Never a sickness that He cannot heal.
Moment by moment in woe or in weal,
Jesus, my Savior, abides with me still."

2

How Can I Have Asthma?

ABOUT a year after my hysterectomy my allergies, which had been an occasional problem for about three years, seemed to be getting worse. My nose started running more and I was doing a lot of sneezing. It seemed to bother me quite a bit especially in the spring when I'd be outside working in our garden.

At first I figured I could handle it, but before long, my allergies became worse. Even though I was never one to take any more pills than I needed, I went to the pharmacy, asked the druggist for something, and for some time took over-the-counter antihistamines. But I never took any more than was absolutely necessary.

A short time later I developed bronchitis. I felt very weak, out of breath, and it was hard for me to do my work. I went to the doctor for a prescription and eventually got over it.

But by the next year, my allergies were a constant problem. It seemed as though I was blowing my nose a lot. My eyes were itchy and I had a scratchy throat. This went on for some time.

Then one night I woke up feeling sick and realized I was wheezing. I figured I must be getting bronchitis again because I'd sounded kind of wheezy when I had it before, so I stayed in bed. I couldn't get back to sleep for quite a while, but the wheezing eventually diminished. By morning I felt much better except for the allergies that always seemed to bother me most early in the day.

Three nights later I felt sick again and once more, I was wheezing. As before, the wheezing and my sickness cleared up by morning and for a few days, everything was fine. But the next night I got so bad I didn't know what to do. Thinking I might feel better where it was cool, I went down to the basement and sat there on the cold tile floor. I thought it might help me breathe a little easier, but it was useless. It didn't help at all.

My allergies and what I began to suspect was asthma instead of bronchitis continued to worsen. One night it was particularly bad, like a nightmare, and I was scared because I'd never experienced anything like it before. I woke Bob and told him I could hardly breathe. Then I sat up in bed until the symptoms weren't quite as bad, praying that they'd never come back. But it happened again a few nights later and then again and again.

After another particularly frightening incident, I went to the pharmacy and bought Bronchaid after I read the label, thinking it would help. But during the next nocturnal attack, I felt even worse after I'd taken the Bronchaid.

That made me realize this was nothing to fool around with. I called an allergist and asked if I could schedule an immediate appointment. Luckily I got in right away. I wasn't wheezing quite as badly but enough for the doctor to confirm what I'd suspected. I had asthma. He immediately ordered a breathing test and said I should be tested for allergies.

"Why am I having these problems at my age? I'm forty-seven and have never had asthma before."

The doctor explained that I wasn't unique. "People can develop allergies and asthma at any age," he said as he handed me a prescription. Again he suggested I take the allergy tests, but I said I'd rather wait and see how the medicine he prescribed worked. Ever an optimist, I figured the prescription would prevent further attacks. I got the prescription filled at the pharmacy on my way home.

After I had been on the medicine for some time, it seemed as though my asthma was getting worse and to top it off, I started feeling nervous. I wondered if it could be the medicine I was taking. I called the allergist's office and explained what was going on. The receptionist told me to come right in, and that day I had the allergy tests. When the doctor came in afterwards, I told him, "I don't know why, but I sure don't feel very well."

He said my tests were positive for grass and tree pollens, ragweed and other weed pollens, house dust, molds, cats, dogs, horses, cattle and hogs, as well as beef, lamb, rye, wheat, cauliflower and broccoli. I had to have allergy shots, he added, explaining that I'd have to come in for a shot every two weeks or else go to a doctor's office or medical center closer to my home. "Just be sure you send the records here when you run low on your solution so we can make up more."

I was leery about going for shots every other week, but on the other hand, having a hard time breathing is not something to mess around with. If the shots would help me feel better, what real choice did I have?

The doctor warned that after a shot, I had to stay in the office for a full twenty minutes just in case I had a reaction. Well, I had reactions, but not the kind he meant. I got nauseated, nausea that sometimes lasted into the next day. And around the site of the injection, my arm itched.

After a few months, my asthma seemed to improve. It wasn't gone, but the attacks were much milder and I thought, "As long as they don't get worse, I can live with this."

I planned everything—vacations, even visits with my mother who lived 280 miles north of us—around the injections because I didn't ever want another bad asthma attack.

For a couple years everything went well. Despite mild bouts of asthma, I felt healthy. So when a wonderful friend of mine suggested catching a bus to Chicago so we could go shopping, I replied, "That sounds like a lot of fun."

The morning of our trip, I woke up early anticipating a fun day. Bob drove me to the mall where I was to meet my friend and two women she knew who were going with us. We boarded the bus at the mall and selected four seats, two on each side of the aisle. In minutes, we were talking, laughing and having a good time. My friend brought a game and we decided we'd play after our first coffee stop.

It was shortly after having coffee and doughnuts that I suddenly started feeling strange—sick to my stomach and with a tightness in my throat that made me feel like I was choking. I felt nervous, too, although whether it was because I'd never felt this way before or because it was some new physical symptom, I couldn't tell. All I knew was that it didn't feel like any flu bug I'd had before.

When my friend asked, "What's wrong?" I replied, "I'm not sure, but I can't play this game right now. I don't feel very well."

They played without me, and once we reached Chicago we stopped to have a good breakfast. Inexplicably, my symptoms disappeared and the rest of the day, I felt fine.

We shopped all day, then boarded the bus for Grand Rapids. Our driver announced where we'd stop for dinner. It sounded good; we were hungry. But as we approached the town where we would eat, once again I felt sick with all the same symptoms.

Although I felt choked up and sick to my stomach, I decided I'd try to eat. Perhaps I was just hungry and needed food. But at the restaurant, nothing on the menu seemed appealing. I ordered anyway and picked at my food while my friends ate.

That night when I got home, I woke Bob and told him I felt really sick and nervous and couldn't understand why. On top of it, my heart was racing. It can't be the allergy shots, I explained. My last one was ten days ago.

He suggested that I try sleeping. I did and after a few minutes, fell soundly asleep.

But after that trip, from time to time the symptoms would recur for no apparent reason. They would last a few hours, during which I was miserable, then disappear. We never were able to figure out why.

3

Calling For an Ambulance

IN 1985, five years after my hysterectomy, I woke from a sound sleep, got out of bed, walked into the kitchen and suddenly felt deathly ill. Nervous. Shaky. Weak. I thought I was going to die.

I called to Bob and asked him to come immediately.

By the time he walked the short distance to the kitchen, I was crying and trembling. I'll never forget the worried, compassionate look on his face. I knew he was scared and that he didn't know what to do.

He could see me shaking, so he sat down and said, "Sit on my lap and tell me what's wrong."

At first, all I could say was, "I'm so sick."

He put my head on his shoulder and told me to relax. Just sit here for a while until you calm down.

"But I need to go to the hospital. Please take me right now."

"Can you just sit here for a little while and calm down?"

"No, please take me," I pleaded.

We sat a few minutes, then I pleaded again, "Please take me." I knew I had to go to the hospital and I would stay there until the doctors could find out what was wrong with me. Something had to be done.

Bob woke our son Rick who was sleeping in the next room, explained where we were going and said we'd be back as soon as possible. He also left a note, just in case Rick wasn't fully awake and didn't remember the conversation the next morning.

I sat in the kitchen while Bob warmed up the car. By the time he returned, got my coat and helped me into it, my heart was racing and I felt so weak and faint that even though I was in my own warm, cozy kitchen, I thought about committing suicide. I clung to Bob as he carried me to the car, wondering if I would ever see my home again.

The ride seemed like it took forever. But finally we pulled up to the emergency area and Bob got a nurse. As she wheeled me into the building, he tried to describe what was wrong but couldn't. Then I tried to explain how I felt and told her I needed something that would make me feel better.

The nurse asked if I could stand up without being dizzy. "No, I'm very dizzy," I replied.

When the doctor came in, he gave me medicine to control the dizziness and ordered some tests. But later, when he came back with the results, he said that even though I appeared to be extremely nervous, everything was normal.

Normal? I was shaking from head to foot! I knew that it was more than just being nervous. And what was there to be nervous about? There was nothing going on in my life to make me nervous. I just felt sick inside and knew with certainty that something awful was wrong.

The doctor gave me pills to make me a little calmer. I took them right away, then sat without moving until they took effect. Later as we drove home, I slipped in and out of a light sleep. I felt better afterwards and in the days that followed, I was calm and able to do my work.

As the days passed, I forgot about that frightening episode. Although I occasionally had a sick spell at night, they were mild and I soon began to believe that those awful nervous attacks had ended. But one night it all came back. I felt as though I had waves of sickness going through my head. Bob and I sat up on the sofa and I kept telling him I was sick. He'd say, "Just stay here, relax. Try to think of something else."

I really did try. But I was sick and extremely nervous. And not knowing why I was having these attacks became a nightmare that would haunt me for several years.

Throughout 1985, the nervous spells continued to occur more and more frequently. In addition, my allergies and asthma seemed to be getting worse even though I was still getting allergy shots.

Then in 1986, I had a really bad asthma attack and when I called my doctor, he told me to come in immediately. By that time I was thoroughly frustrated with the shots. But I kept going to the allergist, reassuring myself that my doctor knew best and that I should follow his advice.

At the doctor's office, I tried to describe how awful I felt. The allergist examined me and ordered the

Spirometry screening a breathing test to see if I had bronchial asthma. It was positive. So he prescribed medication for the asthma, as well as the allergies, and said I should take both. I had to stay on allergy shots, he told me, but I needed a stronger solution. Then he handed me a brown bag of antihistamine samples I could try out when I needed them so I could find out which one worked best.

The medicine he gave me controlled my asthma but it also made my heart beat extremely fast. At the same time, I felt lethargic. I used the medicine only when I had more than a mild asthma attack.

That same year, my bi-weekly shots started to cause repeated reactions. They never occurred while I sat in the waiting room for twenty minutes. Instead I would react three or four hours later and afterwards, during the night, I'd have asthma that would last until morning. One night after the shot my asthma got so bad that nothing helped. The next morning I called the doctor and told him that I'd had a terrible night.

He asked, "How do you feel now?"

"I don't have asthma now, but I'm very weak."

He told me to come in and when I got there, the nurse repeated some of the tests I'd had before.

Frustrated, I asked, "Doctor, why am I having all this trouble now? I've never had asthma in my life and now I'm almost forty-nine."

Again he said people can develop asthma at any stage in their lives. He said it was a bad year for allergies and he was going to change my allergy solution. He put me on a Brethaire inhaler, showing me how to use it, and Proventil for the asthma.

Later, the nurse again demonstrated how to use the inhaler. I told her about my horrible night and how I felt. She was a nice woman and very patient with my attempts to use the inhaler. After trying it a couple times, I told her, "If I need the inhaler badly enough, I'm sure I'll be able to work it."

The doctor returned to remind me that I should call or come in if I had any more problems.

If? It turned out my problems were far from ending. I got even worse as the months went by with colds, sore throats and earaches. For over a year, it seemed as though I was constantly going to my doctor's office for antibiotics and I felt totally run down.

Even so, when a neighbor came over and asked if I'd like to walk with her each evening, I jumped at the chance. We both needed exercise and the companionship sounded good too. She asked when I'd like to start and I replied, "What about tomorrow night?"

Our plan was to start out with a short walk and gradually build up the distance. After a few nights, however, I noticed that I was short of breath. Most nights, after walking, my asthma would bother me. Still, I didn't want to give up the exercise, so even when my neighbor was unable to go, I tried to walk a short distance on my own.

I soon realized I'd be unable to continue going out at night. My heart had started racing I attributed it to all the medication I was on and occasionally, it would skip a beat or two. Then I began having erratic heartbeats—even while I worked around the house.

I told Bob that if it didn't get better, I'd have to call my internist. I'd never had problems with my heart before; something had to be wrong. It wasn't normal for me.

March 1986

A few days later, I scheduled a complete physical exam. My doctor ordered the usual chest X-rays, lab work and other tests. He also wanted me to go to the hospital for a treadmill test.

I'd be so nervous when I was hooked up to the treadmill that I didn't think I'd be able to walk. But God was with me as He has always been each step of the way. He knew how much I could handle.

The doctor told me to keep walking faster and faster until I couldn't walk anymore. It was easy at first, but in no time it became so difficult that I wanted to stop. The doctor told me to keep going so they could get better results. Finally, I just quit and after my heartbeat slowed down, the doctor said everything looked normal.

At first, I was relieved. But then I realized if my heart was normal, then something else had to be wrong. What was causing my problems? Why couldn't I take evening walks anymore? Why was my asthma getting so much worse that I now had attacks almost every evening? And why was my health affecting our social life? Because I didn't feel well, we rarely went out with friends anymore.

I called the doctor again and during the exam told him I didn't feel well at all, that I was nervous and sick. He gave me a complete physical and said, "Everything's normal."

Shortly after the physical, it occurred to me that every time I had an allergy shot, I felt very weak afterwards. It became obvious the week Bob and I were getting ready to take a short trip. The day before we were supposed to leave, I completed all but the last-minute packing, then went for my shot. The next morning I felt terrible—extremely tired, weak and out of breath. I told Bob I couldn't help pack the car; it was up to him. "I think I may be getting the flu," I explained, but as soon as the words were out of my mouth, I realized that it wasn't likely that I had the flu. The symptoms were more likely related to the shot I'd had the day before. We went anyway and I felt ill the whole time we were gone, even though the shortness of breath and weakness disappeared after two days.

I had never liked the idea of having shots; now, more than ever, the thought of having one frightened me. After a shot, my nights were nightmares, so much so that occasionally I'd have to sit up in a chair throughout the night.

After one bad night, shortly after Bob left for work, I sat at the table, trying to drink a cup of coffee. I really wanted to sleep, but I figured if I did, I'd probably be up all the next night. So instead of going back to bed that morning, I prayed, as I had so many other times, asking for God's help and intervention. I prayed that He would give me some relief from my asthma attacks, but I was full of doubt. I didn't realize

God would eventually answer my prayers as He always does.

It was hot that morning and I remember thinking about what to eat. I had to be careful about what I ate because now milk products didn't agree with me. I preferred to drink hot juice because it always went down much better than milk unless I was having an asthma attack.

I tuned the radio to my favorite station and heard a forecast for a very hot sticky day. Then, the station played some of my favorite songs. Afterwards, I heard an advertisement for a health food store.

"Do you suffer from allergies?" a woman's voice asked. "Are you allergic to certain products? Come in to see me. My advice is free."

I could feel excitement building. Was this an answer to my prayer? Sitting alone in the house, I prayed again. "I have a need, dear God. What must I do? Give me an answer, please."

I thought about the ad, wondering how health foods could possibly affect allergies. But still, something was telling me to listen. It seemed to me that God was saying, "Go. Go see her."

Finishing my coffee, I decided I had to try something different. My allergies and asthma were worse, not better, despite all the shots I'd had and medication I'd taken.

I gathered up all my pills and the inhaler, put them in a brown paper bag and thought, "Here goes." Despite my wheezing and the humid air that seemed to make it worse, I climbed in the car and headed for the health food store.

4

Treating Myself

January 1986

I was still wheezing when I walked into the store a short time later and nervously asked the clerk, a young man, whom I should see about allergies and asthma. He was very polite and asked me to wait while he got the nutritionist, a woman named Pat who owned the store. She came out almost immediately and sat down at a huge desk with rows of books behind her.

I was impressed. "If she has all those books," I thought, "she must be really smart and know what she's doing."

"Have a chair. Sit down and relax," she said, a friendly smile on her face.

I needed a chair. I was very tired.

"I'm here because I have allergies and asthma very bad," I told her, my voice crackling with emotion. The words poured out. "I don't know what to do. The medication I'm taking doesn't help and when I do take it, I feel worse. My heart beats so fast sometimes I get scared. And I'm scared of the asthma medication. Sometimes I think I'm going to die. The shots are not helping one bit; in fact, I'm always getting reactions to the shots. And lately I have been getting weak and short of breath."

"I can't go on like this," I sobbed. "I have to do something. Can something be done?"

"I had a woman come in here not too long ago who had asthma and hers is almost gone," the nutritionist replied.

My heart leaped at her words. "Oh, dear God," I prayed, "could this please happen to me. I wouldn't know how to act if my asthma would leave me. I could never thank You enough."

But what if this isn't God's plan for me? Maybe I really do have some bad illness. Maybe His plan is that I gradually die. Hope and fear made my head whirl as I pulled the medicine out of the bag to show the nutritionist what I was taking.

"Your problem seems to be mostly in your respiratory tract so we'll try to treat that first," she said, taking out a notebook and writing down a nutritional diet with vitamins and supplements and some foods I should avoid. Then she took three bottles of vitamins off the shelf and explained when and how I should take them.

"I'll do whatever you say. I'm at your mercy," I told her gratefully, not once thinking to ask how much it would cost. Money didn't seem important. I'd already spent a lot of money on different drugs and allergy shots and hadn't gotten any relief. Besides, when you're as sick as I was, money's not the object. I wasn't at all concerned about the cost.

We talked a little longer, then I left thanking her for taking time to talk to me. I closed the door feeling relieved and somehow lighter. But I also had strong doubts that the vitamins could be effective.

Shrugging my shoulders, I thought, "It's worth a try." Wanting to believe a miracle could take place, I offered another silent prayer.

"Dear God, can this help me? Thou only knowest if it can. And You can do all things."

Even if I only got partial relief, I decided, I would be thankful to God. And whatever happened, I vowed, I'd let the nutritionist know whether her vitamins had worked.

When I got home, I took the first vitamins. I could barely contain my excitement. I wanted so much to talk to Bob immediately and tell him what I had done. As always, he supported my decision to try something new. "It might bring relief and even if it doesn't," he said, "you can always stop taking them."

I worried that my stomach might not tolerate large doses of vitamins, but I had no problems. After two months of taking them, I began to think they actually were giving me some relief. Six months later, I was positive they worked. It was time to get off the allergy shots, I decided. But when I called the allergist's office and told the nurse I did not plan to come in any more, in a stern voice, she warned, "You'd better not stop taking the shots!"

I didn't say another word. Hanging up the phone, I thought, "I'll just go to a different allergist if I need allergy shots again." Little did I realize that within a year, I'd seriously reconsider getting the shots, anything to improve how I felt.

March 13, 1987

I was having a bad day and in desperation, I decided to go back to an allergist. "Maybe I'm feeling sick and nervous because I went off the allergy shots," I reasoned. "Maybe I should have stayed on them longer."

Knowing I couldn't go back to the first allergist, I grabbed the phone book and looked for another. Then I called and asked if I could come in right away because I felt so nervous. The sympathetic receptionist scheduled me right in.

The allergist said he'd like to run the allergy tests all over again. After the testing, he told me, "You don't need shots, but I'll give you some medication you can take when your allergies get bad."

I was relieved and told him I didn't think I needed allergy shots any more because of the vitamins I was taking.

He asked what they were and when I told him, he said, "Vitamin A will make you funny in the head."

"Oh, no," I thought, "is this what is giving me thoughts of suicide and making me sick and nervous?"

I seriously debated whether I should heed his warning, but the vitamins won. How could I ignore the fact that my allergies and asthma were constantly getting better. And even though I was nervous, I rarely had to take any of the nine allergy or two asthma medications that had been prescribed at one time or another. God had answered that prayer, I decided. Perhaps in His goodness, He will decide to help me again.

5

What's Wrong With Me, Doctor?

March 27, 1987

IT started like any other day. When I got out of bed, I made myself a cup of coffee while Bob took a shower. Then I packed his lunch and made him coffee and toast. We watched the news for a while, then he left for work and I was alone.

About an hour later, I decided to do the laundry. I was sorting clothes in the basement when I started feeling faint, then dizzy and extremely sick. I had no strength except for my heart which was pounding so hard that I was sure I was having a heart attack. I started crying and shaking at the same time. I didn't know what to do. I didn't think I could make it upstairs but somehow I managed to crawl up the stairs and to the phone.

When an ambulance arrived about five minutes later, I could hardly talk because I was trembling so much and was extremely nervous. I insisted that the attendants call Bob at work before they took me to the hospital, I wanted him by my side.

I'll never forget that ride to the hospital. Nauseated, I clung desperately to the pan the medical attendant gave me. He sat by my side all the time asking if I was OK. I wasn't OK. I really didn't think I'd live through the ten minutes it took to get to the hospital.

When we arrived, I saw Bob standing at the emergency room door with a strained, worried look on his face. He and a nurse helped me into a wheelchair and pushed me into one of the emergency room cubicles. The doctor came in a short time later and I tried to explain what had happened. It was difficult. How could I really explain how awful I felt, how sick I was?

The doctor ordered blood tests and an EKG to see if I was having a heart attack, then he left Bob and me alone. Frightened, I pleaded with Bob to call the doctor back because I was dying. He kept reassuring me that I'd be all right, but I wasn't. I was terribly sick and agitated and eventually someone gave me medication to calm me down. Some time later, a nurse walked into the examining room and told me I'd be all right. She asked if I could sit up.

"Yes," I said, sitting up. Then I got to my feet.

When the doctor came back, he talked to Bob about how nervous I was and told him to take me to *my* doctor that same day. He asked a few questions, then he pointedly asked Bob what he had done to me. Poor Bob. To think that anyone would suspect him of abusing his wife!

On the way home I felt much calmer, but as we neared the house and pulled into the driveway, I became apprehensive again. I was frightened I might not be able to climb the stairs and get into the house. Why was it that something as comforting as coming home had now turned into a nightmare?

As I laboriously climbed the stairs, with each step I tightly gripped the railing. I knew I would fall if I didn't hang on. Climbing those few steps took forever and once indoors, I realized I was drained and needed to lie down. Although the sick feeling had disappeared, I still felt very weak and shaky. My heart was beating fast and I could hardly talk. While I rested, Bob called my physician and made an appointment for later that day.

At the doctor's office that afternoon, Bob helped me to a chair, then went to talk to the nurse. I had just settled down when I realized some of my friends were in the waiting room too.

"Oh, no," I thought. "I'm too nervous and sick to talk to them."

They came right over and sat beside me. I could barely speak, but I tried to explain that I was really sick. My friend thought it might be the flu and while she chatted happily, I silently prayed, "Nurse, please call me in right now. I'm too sick to sit here and talk." My friend did not notice the stress I was under as I waited to hear my name.

Eventually, it was my turn and when the doctor came into the examining room, he asked if I'd had a bad day. I was so choked up that I could only respond with a weak, "Yes." He ordered some lab tests: a urine analysis, blood tests, chest X-rays and a tetanus shot. The results were normal, essentially the same as those of the year before when I had had my complete physical. After checking me over, my physician said he couldn't find anything wrong.

I asked the doctor if he'd prescribe something for my nerves. He said he would and told the nurse to give me some samples so I could start immediately. The first pill didn't help at all. About four hours later, following the doctor's instructions, I took another. Then I tried to eat dinner, but I couldn't get anything down. I was feeling ill again.

After we cleared up the kitchen, Bob asked if I'd mind if he went to our son's house. He'd promised to help with some redecorating.

"Please don't go," I replied. "I can't be here alone."

"I won't be too long and you can call me if you need me."

Reluctantly, I agreed, but I warned Bob I might have to go to the hospital. Luckily another one of our sons, Doug, came and sat with me while Bob was gone.

I managed to get through the next two days and nights feeling not quite sick, but not well either. Something was still wrong.

March 30, 1987

Three days after my trip to the emergency room, I became deathly ill and once again it occurred about three hours after Bob left for work. Again, thoughts of suicide entered my mind. Fighting panic, I got to the phone, called Bob and asked him to come home immediately. Fortunately, he did.

I always felt better when Bob was with me. It was comforting to know that if I really got sick, he'd be there to take care of me. But it wasn't realistic for him to be there every day. He couldn't be at home with me, not if he wanted to keep his job.

I had scheduled another physical exam for April 3. If only I can hold off for a few days, I told myself, the doctor is sure to discover what's wrong with me. But those four days were a nightmare, some days worse than others.

April 3, 1987

At the doctor's office, I again complained about how I felt. "Doctor, I'm so nervous and sick. What can be wrong?"

After examining me, he told me I had a serious respiratory infection. He put me on antibiotics and gave me a sample to take immediately.

"Maybe this is what's causing my dizziness and weakness," I thought.

Then I told him the nerve medication he'd given me didn't work and asked for something else. He hesitated long enough that I knew he didn't want to put me on anything else.

"Doctor, I need something really bad," I pleaded, thinking, "If only you had my body and could experience what I'm feeling, then you'd know. You'd find something to make it better."

He finally agreed to try something different and walking to the door, he repeated, "Everything looks good."

I knew the nurse quite well because she had been giving me my allergy shots. So as I got ready to leave, I told her that I needed something for my nerves. She showed me the medication the doctor had prescribed and assured me it would make me feel better.

I wanted to be optimistic, but once I got home in that empty house, I was anything but hopeful. When I was alone, I continually replayed the script that constantly ran through my head: "I am getting progressively worse day by day," I'd tell myself. "Why can't they find out what is wrong with me? Am I ever going to get better?"

By lunchtime, I could feel the antibiotic starting to work. But it was also making me feel sick. I debated whether I should eat. "Some toast shouldn't hurt," I thought. I fixed it, but even without butter, I could not get it down. I had reached the stage that most of the time, even the thought of food nauseated me.

By 3:30 p.m., I felt physically weak and emotionally ill. The new medication for my nerves hadn't made a difference and I had to sit by myself for five more hours because Bob had to work late that day.

"Five more hours! I can't wait that long," I decided, trying to calm the panic that was starting to overwhelm me. "I have to do something. Maybe the medical center near our house can give me something that can help."

I drove there, parked and sat in my car for quite a while thinking that the pill I'd taken would wear off at any moment. I kept crying and asking God what

I must do. But my thoughts turned to suicide and I knew I had to get indoors.

I walked inside and the receptionist said the doctor could see me right away. "How wonderful," I thought. "I don't have to wait."

As the doctor examined me, I told him about the medication. "If the medicine is causing the reaction," he said, "it will probably take a few more hours to wear off." He suggested I sit in the waiting room until I felt better.

I didn't move. I remember thinking, "Surely he can see my quivering lips and hear it in my voice even if he doesn't know how I feel inside. I'm sick! Why can't anyone see that and help me?"

Again he suggested I sit in the waiting room, so I went there and asked the receptionist to call Bob. I wanted to tell him where I was, that I was OKand that he didn't have to leave work or worry about me. My poor husband! By then his life was in constant upheaval. He never knew what to expect.

As for me, despite my frayed nerves, at the moment I felt relieved just knowing I was sitting in the medical center and was near a doctor. If anything happened, I'd get instant care. I sat there for about two hours before leaving for home.

Bob and our son Rick were waiting in the kitchen when I returned. They looked sad and I knew they didn't know what to say. I knew they were concerned about my health and that they felt helpless, too.

Bob asked, "Are you hungry?"

"I probably should eat something, but not too much because I haven't been eating hardly at all."

"How does a *Burger King* sound?"

"It sounds pretty good," I replied. Already I felt better because the people I loved were beside me. Being alone all the time gave me too much time to think, to worry about what was wrong and wonder if I'd ever get well.

Later when Bob handed me the burger, it took a concentrated effort and almost forty-five minutes for me to eat it. I could only nibble off one small piece at a time because my throat felt choked up. And even then, I needed the distraction of television to chew and swallow.

A few hours later, I felt sick again and headed for bed thinking I might be able to sleep it off. Sleep didn't help, nor did the nerve pill I took. I had a miserable night and by morning, I felt even worse. My nerves were frayed, so the pill hadn't worked at all. I wondered if the pill compounded my symptoms and whether the antibiotic I was taking added to the reaction.

I debated what to do. It was Saturday, but early, and I knew my doctor's office would be open until noon. Perhaps I should ask whether I really needed to take the antibiotic. And if the doctor examined me again, maybe this time something would show up, some tangible evidence of how I felt. If he found something, then he could give me the right medication and then I would actually get better.

Luckily Bob was working outdoors. If he knew what I was up to, he wouldn't like it. He'd question whether it was wise to go to all these doctors, so I decided I wouldn't tell him what I planned to do.

Within fifteen minutes I was on the phone asking the receptionist if I could come in that morning. When she asked why, I told her that I needed to know if I still needed antibiotics for my infection. I got choked up when I tried to describe how I felt. It was embarrassing to tell her the same old things I'd said before. She said my doctor wasn't in, but if I was willing to see another, I could come in at 10 a.m.

I made the appointment and headed for the yard where I told Bob I had to run an errand. He looked at me kind of funny. He knew I didn't usually run off on errands by myself, so he asked what I had to do. I started crying and told him the truth. I think that morning Bob realized that I really was very sick.

All the way to the doctor's office I pictured their reaction, "Her again!"

"If only they could live through just one day of what I am experiencing," I thought, "they'd understand."

As soon as I arrived, the nurse called me in and after the doctor examined me, he said I didn't need any more antibiotics. He was about to leave the examining room when I hesitantly asked him if I could have a different kind of nerve pill. "I need something that will work," I said.

"I think you should go on an anti-depressant for a while," he replied.

Anti-depressants? Another pill? What was happening to me—a woman who rarely even took aspirin for a headache? I told the doctor I'd rather wait and see if it was really necessary.

As the nurse walked me to the desk, I played on her sympathy. "The nerve pill doesn't work. I need something that really works." She promised to get the doctor to prescribe something, went into his office and a short time later, came out with a prescription. She called the pharmacy so I could pick it up on my way home. I managed to take those new pills for two days. Then I called the nurse, told her they didn't work either and that I didn't want to take them anymore.

By this time, I had tried out three different pills for nerves and nothing worked! I was beginning to think I had an incurable illness.

On three occasions during the next few weeks, I found myself sitting in the medical center parking lot. Oddly I found it comforting to know I could walk in any second if my condition became unbearable. It was better than being alone in an empty house, I rationalized.

Most days, I ate only a little food. I was losing weight. But even worse, I started canceling appointments.

On April 10, we had plans to go out to dinner with friends, but I called and made excuses that I was sick. What else could I say? "I'll call when I feel better," I promised. But I didn't really mean it. I didn't want to see friends or my family and I didn't want them to come to our house to visit.

April 13, 1987

Bob answered the phone. It was my mother. She spoke to Bob a few minutes, then asked about me.

He came to the family room where I was resting on the couch and said, “Can you talk to your mother?”

I refused despite the fact that she was calling long distance. Bob walked back to the phone very slowly and said, “She's sick and can't talk.”

My mother hadn't been told about my hospital visit because we didn't want her to worry. But that night Bob filled her in, without going into great detail. He said I was very nervous. Then he came back to me and said, “Your mother would like to come down this weekend.”

“Oh, tell her I can't have her,” I blurted out. The thought of a visit made me more agitated. I didn't want to be unkind or hurt my mother. It was difficult to refuse a visit because we'd always been great friends, but I felt I couldn't talk to her or see her right now.

I asked God to help my very dear mother understand and told Bob to tell her that I'd write if I could.

Later, in a very loving letter, I tried to explain what I was going through. “Mother, I hope and pray that some day I can make this all up to you.”

In reply, she wrote that she felt bad that this was happening to me and that I was constantly in her prayers.

I made other vows that night, too. I vowed that when God delivered me from this nightmare I would repay my family and friends for their kindness and understanding. I know that God sends us trials and that they are all for one reason: to draw us closer to Him. I knew I could not give up on God and that even on days when it was hard to pray, I had to keep on praying. And I did. I had faith that someday He would answer my prayers.

A few days after mother called, I became suicidal. Even though it was Sunday, I got on the phone and called my physician.

"Is there anything I can take," I asked the doctor answering calls that weekend. "I'm so weak and nervous."

He snapped back, "Just try to relax and don't worry about things. Take it easy!"

I crumbled and tried to pray. "Dear Lord. When the doctors can't do any more, will You do Your best work?"

But I got no relief talking to Him. Before He answered my prayers, I had to let God take total control of me and my illness.

April 16, 1987

I was resting on the family–room sofa when I heard a car pull into the driveway. Bob looked out the window and said, "It's the kids."

I really wanted to see our dear son, his wife and our only grandchild, but my illness kept me away.

"Oh, no. Please go out and tell them I don't feel well. Tell them to come another time."

Bob couldn't do that. He went outdoors to greet them and told them I didn't feel well. While they were still talking outside, I got up, walked to the bedroom and shut the door. Not only was I unable to talk, but I also didn't want them to see me. I knew with all the weight I had lost I looked awful.

Shortly after they got indoors, I heard a knock on the door.

"Oh, no," I thought. "God help me through this. Help me talk." Despite my misgivings, I opened the door, came out and managed to get through the visit. I was glad Bob hadn't heeded my plea to send them away. I was genuinely happy to see them, especially our dear grandson.

Again I prayed that the day would soon come when I would be able to fully explain to everyone what I was feeling and assure them that I'd never fake anything just to avoid their company.

April 26, 1987

I called the doctor again and told the receptionist I had to come in. I could no longer walk without desperately hanging onto furniture, anything that would keep me from falling down.

"Can you come in around 2 p.m.?" she asked.

"Yes," I promised, knowing the drive would not be easy. "I have to come in."

The doctor I had seen three weeks earlier examined me and said, "You have a choice. You can either see a psychiatrist or I will put you on an anti-depressant."

I agreed to take the anti-depressant. "Maybe it's the answer," I thought as I drove home.

When Bob got to the house that night, I explained that I'd gone to the doctor and that he'd given me an anti-depressant. "Will you go to the pharmacy for me?"

Bob got my prescription filled and I took the first dose that evening. Three pills later, I was so weak and sick that I could not get off the sofa. I called out to Bob who was working in the yard.

"Something's happening to me. I'm so sick."

He called the doctor's office and told the nurse what was happening. "Tell your wife she should immediately stop taking them," she said.

Take another? No way! I wouldn't want to go through that again.

Each day was a nightmare and I really believed I'd eventually be taken to the hospital and would never get out.

May 7, 1987

I'd reached the end of my rope. I knew the doctors were tired of hearing my voice, but in desperation, I called again and asked for something to make me feel better.

The nurse scheduled an appointment with the internist who would be seeing patients the next afternoon and said I should bring with me all the medication I was taking.

"The vitamins, too?"

"Everything," she replied. "We're going to run some blood tests."

"Good, because there's something terribly wrong. I'll do whatever it takes."

Dreading the thought of being alone in the house because by then I feared I was losing my mind, I asked the nurse if it would be all right to come in early and sit in the waiting room until my afternoon appointment. She said it would be no problem, so the next morning, I scooped my three vitamins and the allergy and asthma pills I had kept "just in case," put them in a brown paper sack and headed off to the doctor's office.

In the examining room later, I placed the medicine on the examining table as the nurse instructed. When the doctor came in, he asked, "Are you anxious?"

"Yes, and then some."

He examined me, then looked at the pill bottles, asking how often and how much I took of each. Then he said, "Get rid of this vitamin and that vitamin and the Vitamin C."

"I need Vitamin C," I protested.

"Well, at least cut way down!"

Without mentioning the allergy and asthma medications, he said, "We'll let you know how the blood tests turn out." Then he left the room.

I was frustrated and unhappy, but desperate too. Trying to look at the bright side, I thought, "Perhaps the vitamins are giving me all this trouble."

I could be reacting to a poison in my system caused by excessive vitamins or something similar, the nurse said, suggesting that I drink plenty of water to flush out the poison. So I went home and started drinking, glass after glass after glass. I also stopped taking the vitamins for a few days because I wanted to hear from the doctor's office before I took any more.

For three long days I waited to hear about the tests, then I got impatient and wanted to know the results.

I called the doctor's office and after a five-minute delay, the nurse told me all the tests were normal.

My heart skipped a beat. How could I be cured if they still didn't know what was wrong?

"Can I take the vitamins," I asked.

The nurse hesitated, then answered, "Yes."

I knew the doctor didn't want me to take them, but the nutritionist had said I needed them. They had helped so much with my allergies and asthma that I didn't want to stop taking them. "If they made me sick, then I'll stop," I decided. "Until then I'll go back to my usual dose."

I don't know how I managed to get through the next week except that I believe God was listening and was with me every step of the way.

That week we were blessed with the birth of another grandchild. I was overjoyed, but despite my happiness, I couldn't go to see the new baby and the others in my son's family.

One day was particularly bad. I remember it because that was the day I heard an ad on the radio saying a medical supply store was doing free health screens that day, blood pressure, pulse rates, blood sugar, cholesterol, hearing and eyesight.

It was already 4:30 p.m., but I still had time to get there if I hurried. So I hopped in the car and luckily found a parking spot as soon as I pulled into the lot. I rushed into line minutes before closing and chatted with the woman ahead of me while we waited to be tested. This time there was no delay in getting the results. At every station, it was the same report—normal. I went home with a heavy heart and still, no answers.

Another weekend went by and on Monday, Bob went to work. After having had him home all weekend, I didn't want him to leave. He had been gone for only an hour when I became overwhelmed with anxiety. I simply couldn't be alone in the house. Again, the thought of suicide filled my head; so of course, normal activities like sitting, sleeping and eating were out of the question.

I decided to call Bob and tell him to come home immediately, no matter what his boss or co-workers thought. But when I asked for him, one of them said, "I'll find him if I can and have him call."

Desperately, I prayed and asked God to answer my prayers that my husband would call and then come home. I was still wiping tears from my eyes when the phone rang. It was Bob.

"Please come home right away," I pleaded.

He hesitated and I felt guilty that I'd even had to ask such a favor. I've always been extremely independent and never asked anyone for anything. Before I got sick, I'd never asked Bob to come home from work. But this was different. I was on the verge of committing suicide and I needed him.

"Come right now," I demanded, and as I started to hang up the phone, I heard him say, "OK."

It wasn't that Bob didn't want to help me; he had to think about his job. What must his boss be saying, let alone thinking? I felt guilty and wished again that my health would return. But right now my life was at stake.

When Bob drove up about ten minutes later, I met him at the door crying, shaking and barely able to stand. As we hugged, he asked, "What's wrong?"

"Don't leave me here alone. I can't be here alone."

"I can't take the day off," he said, but he said it in a loving way. Deep inside I knew he was right, but even so, I pleaded, "Don't leave me."

We were silent for a long time. Then I said, "I don't know what to do. I'm so sick."

He tried to comfort me and that calmed my fears a little. Then he said, "Why don't you get your coat on and come with me?"

"I can't do that."

"Why can't you?"

I didn't reply for a minute or two, but he kept repeating, "Come on. I can't take off from work."

I protested, "I'm too sick."

"Come on. This will help you get your mind off things."

I had to admit that going with him would be better than being in the house alone. Still I asked, "What will the guys who work with you think?"

"I'll tell you what," he replied. "I'll go do some different work today so you won't see anyone. But first, let's go out and have coffee and something to eat."

When I said I couldn't eat anything, he said, "Then just have some coffee."

That sounded better, so I said I'd get my coat. Because I was self conscious and embarrassed about what people were thinking about me, I worried about running into anyone we knew. But fortunately, we didn't know anyone at the coffee shop. Bob ordered breakfast with coffee and I said I'd just have a few sips from his cup. I simply didn't have an appetite and even if I was hungry, couldn't swallow much food.

While we sat there, Bob asked, "Do you feel better now?"

"A little bit," I replied, not mentioning how I hurt and the turmoil I felt inside.

Bob finished his breakfast and suggested we get on our way. I reluctantly agreed. To be honest, I really didn't want to go anywhere. Most of the time, I just wanted to curl up and die. But if someone was with me, especially Bob, I was distracted and that gave me some relief even though it only lasted a short while.

We climbed into Bob's truck and headed for some railroad tracks he had to check out. As we drove, he said he didn't think anyone from the office would be there.

"I hope not," I declared. The thought that anyone would see me riding in Bob's truck made me uncomfortable and embarrassed.

Bob checked signal switches and the flashing lights at two railroad crossings to see if they were in working order. Then at his third stop, we saw one of the crew heading toward us in his truck.

"Oh, no! Is he coming here? I don't want him to see me," I cried out. I felt so ashamed that Bob had to take me with him to work despite the fact that it was the first time in all the years we'd been married.

I knew I didn't have a choice, but even so, I didn't want to be seen.

"I'm going to duck down so he won't see me," I told Bob.

The man never did come near our truck, but he was close enough that I'm sure he would have spotted me if I'd been sitting up straight. I stayed hunched down until the coast was clear. From that point on, I constantly searched every direction to make sure we wouldn't run into anyone else. It was a long trying day, but ironically, it helped keep my mind off my problems.

An hour before quitting time, Bob's boss radioed the truck that there was track trouble and Bob should go to the site. So instead of getting off work at 5 p.m. as usual, he worked until 6. I didn't complain. I had my husband at my side and I needed that security.

May 15, 1987

Crying, choking, every part of my body nervous and trembling, I called the internist's office and pleaded, "Please take me in."

The receptionist said I should come in immediately.

I felt embarrassed and ashamed to be back so soon. When I saw the doctor, I told him the same story as before. "I'm so extremely nervous that I can't go on for another day."

"Hold your hands up and close your eyes," he said, wanting to see how much I was shaking.

I started crying again, tears coursing down my cheeks. "I only want to get better."

"There is nothing that I can do," he replied. "I want you to go see a psychiatrist. He will help you. I'll have the nurse come in and she will set up an appointment."

The nurse called a psychiatrist associated with a mental hospital. "The doctor can see you in a week," she told me.

My throat choked up even tighter. My thoughts were a jumble; a mental hospital! This was the worst blow I had yet received. Am I that bad? What is going to happen to me now? Where will I have to go? Will I ever come out of the hospital if I have to go there? Will I ever see my grandchildren and my family again?

"I can't wait a week. That's too long," I blurted out. "I need to see someone right now."

When the nurse asked if I wanted to call a psychiatrist, I replied weakly, "I'll try." I don't know how I managed to drive home that day because of my trembling. I only know God was one step ahead of me all the way.

6

Am I Crazy?

ONCE I got home, I leafed through the yellow pages looking for a psychiatrist. I picked one out and dialed the number. When the receptionist answered, I told her I needed to see someone right away. She said she had an opening that afternoon.

"I'll try to make it."

I hung up, then called Bob to tell him I had to go to a psychiatrist and that I'd found one who could see me right away. "Can you take me there?"

"No, I really can't take off from work."

Deep down I knew Bob was right because of all the days he'd missed while sitting home with me. But I begged anyway. "I'm so shaky I don't know if I can drive. I don't want to have an accident."

"Arlene, I can't. You know that."

I kept begging, but after he said no several more times, I reluctantly conceded, "Ok, I'll try to go by myself."

I stepped outdoors into brilliant sunshine, but it failed to lift my mood. I sat at the patio table and prayed. If ever I needed God's help, it was now.

"Please God, spare my life so I can see the psychiatrist and in Your bountiful mercy, let him help me."

A few hours later I climbed into the car even though I knew I was too sick to drive for five minutes, let alone all the way to the psychiatrist's office. But God was with me that afternoon. I arrived safely.

Sitting in the waiting room, I wondered if anyone was staring at me. I knew I looked awful. I'd lost more than ten pounds and rarely bothered to fix my hair or wear makeup. Self-consciously, I reached for a magazine, but I couldn't pick it up! My body was shaking so much that I couldn't control my fingers. My lips were also trembling and when I had talked to the receptionist, my voice had quivered. It even seemed as if I was shaking inside.

"If only I could end it all," I thought. But I could hear God saying, "Be patient."

Every time the door opened, I looked up hopefully. I was impatient. I wanted to get into the doctor's office because I couldn't control my shaking. But as it turned out, I was one of the last patients to be seen that afternoon.

When the doctor finally called my name, as we walked to his office, he asked, "How are you?"

"I don't feel well. I'm terribly nervous," I replied tersely. I couldn't trust my voice, so I didn't want to elaborate. I sat down in a huge leather chair and for a few minutes, the doctor chatted about the weather to make me feel comfortable. Then he asked about my family.

Dismayed, I thought, "I'm not here because of family problems. I'm here because I'm shaking and suicidal! It has nothing to do with my family. We love each other. We're close to our children and I've always been happy and lived life to its fullest."

So why was I here? How could I make the psychiatrist see that my family had nothing to do with my problems? I came to the psychiatrist because my doctor gave me no choice; he told me I had to go. I forced myself to answer the psychiatrist's questions. I had to reply because he was only trying to help and I would do anything if it would make me feel better.

We talked for about ten minutes and at the end of the conversation, the doctor said he wanted me to take the tranquilizer Xanax and an anti-depressant called Sinequan. I had to take both of them three times a day.

"I've had three different kinds of nerve pills and two made me feel worse, more hyperactive. The anti-depressant made me so terribly sick and weak that I couldn't get off the sofa. What will these medicines do to me? Will they do the same thing?"

"You should have no side effects," he answered, "but it may take a few days for your body to adjust to them. I want you to go straight to the pharmacy and take the Xanax right away."

"I will," I promised. "I simply can't go on the way I am now."

Before I left, I asked if I could attend a wedding the next day. He advised me to take it easy. He knew the Sinequan was going to make me feel awful until my system adjusted to it, but he didn't tell me that.

As I left the office, I made an appointment for June 5, a month away, then stopped at the pharmacy on my way home and immediately swallowed a Xanax. It calmed me down a little, but the Sinequan I took later made me sick and weak.

"I have to bear it," I rationalized. "Eventually the pills will take effect and I'll feel better."

The next morning I knew for certain we'd have to skip the wedding. Bob called our friends to say I was sick and we'd be unable to attend. I wouldn't let him say anything else because I was too ashamed to admit I'd been to a psychiatrist. What would they think?

No one outside our immediate family knew what was happening to me and even our sons knew very little. Even so, our friends may have guessed I was extremely ill. They probably thought I was going off the deep end.

About a week later, I still felt awful so I called the psychiatrist. He said my body would have to adjust to the medicine and that I should be patient. The Xanax did keep my nerves under control but that first month was rough.

June 5, 1987

A month later, I was sitting in the psychiatrist's waiting room again. I felt only a bit more comfortable than on my first visit. I wasn't quite as shaky and weak, but I still couldn't leaf through a magazine while I waited. After the doctor called me in, we talked for a few minutes, then he asked how the medication was working.

"Better. I don't feel quite so weak."

We chatted until my fifteen minutes were up, then he wrote prescriptions for the next month's supply. On the way out I paid $45 for the visit and made an appointment for July 2.

"Dear God, I hope this will work," I prayed. "Something has to work soon."

The next month was almost as trying as the first, but I faithfully took the pills always hoping they'd make me feel better.

In July, the psychiatrist talked about visiting Chicago. He liked to go there as much as Bob and I do. Then he wrote out prescriptions which would take me through July to my early August appointment. Once again we chatted for fifteen minutes and on my way out, I paid the bill and made an appointment for four weeks later.

In mid-July, when I'd been on Xanax and Sinequan for about two and a half months, we got an invitation to an anniversary party for close friends. Bob wanted to go, but I knew it was impossible because I wouldn't be able to talk to all our friends who would be there. But what could we tell the couple? When a mutual friend called to ask if we were going, I stammered, "No, I don't feel well." I was embarrassed that she had mentioned the party but also upset that she had forced me into making excuses that sounded hollow even to me. If I'd been healthy, I knew, I'd have had little patience listening to someone who kept repeating the same old thing.

"Dear God, make them understand," I prayed. "If they really knew how nervous I am, they wouldn't ask me all these questions."

The week of the party we sent our friends a nice gift-spending more than we would have under ordinary circumstances—and a card that again expressed our regrets that we couldn't be there. Once again I prayed, "Dear God, make them understand that we wouldn't stay away on purpose. We love them dearly."

In August I made an effort to go out with Bob occasionally because he liked going out and having fun. It wasn't fair to punish him by having him sit home day after day with an invalid wife. I didn't want to tie him down like that, but I couldn't help it. If Bob weren't such a patient, understanding man, by then surely we would have had deep rifts in our marriage. I don't like to think about what might have occurred had I had a different husband.

Early in October, even though I still felt weak and gripped the railing whenever I went downstairs to keep from falling, it seemed as though my nerves were getting more under control. Another positive sign was that food actually started tasting good and I was eating more than before. But I still avoided talking to people.

Nevertheless I was encouraged. I had only four more visits with the psychiatrist. Surely by the time they ended, and after I'd been on Xanax and Sinequan for nine months, I'd feel more like myself.

In October, the psychiatrist asked how I was doing and I replied, "Better. I'm sleeping well, but why do I still feel so nervous?"

He avoided giving me a definite answer. "It could be a number of things."

I persisted. "I don't have anything to be nervous about. We have three lovely sons who never gave us any trouble and two darling grandchildren. My mother—and some other women—think I'm feeling like this because of my hysterectomy and change of life. Can they be right?"

"No," he replied. Then as my fifteen minutes drew to a close, he wrote prescriptions for another month's supply of pills and said he'd see me next month.

Even though I took the Sinequan religiously, I was certain I didn't need an anti-depressant. Depressed? I don't think I've ever been depressed. In fact people usually said I was one of the happiest people they knew and I'd never disagreed. How could I? God had always been wonderful to me. Until 1985, I'd had good health. I'd had a happy childhood, loving parents who taught me to love God, my parents and my grandparents, and now I have a loving husband. How could I be depressed, and if so, about what?

But how could I argue with the doctor? They have all that education and know so much more than I do. So I continued to do exactly as I was told and never missed one pill.

One day my mother called and asked how I was feeling. "Better, mother."

"That's good. You do exactly what the doctor says. Take the pills when you're supposed to."

"I do. I want to get better," I replied.

"I know you do. I'm praying for you every day. I pray that you will soon be well again."

I don't know why her comment made me choke up, but I started to cry and then I became more nervous. If I needed proof that I still had a long way to go before I'd actually be well, there it was.

I continued to go out with Bob, but it wasn't easy. I still didn't want to see people, but when friends called, I'd force myself to be social. I couldn't always say no.

One evening my mother phoned and asked when we'd be coming up north for a visit.

"Perhaps we can come up this weekend," I said, feeling guilty about the excuses I'd made in the past. Mother was so pleased when she heard my reply that, simply out of guilt, I forced down my irritation at having been trapped into taking a trip I didn't want to make in the first place.

Despite being nervous about being so far from home, the visit went well and as we got ready to leave, mother said she'd like to come to Grand Rapids so we could have more time to catch up on everything. Reluctantly I agreed, telling myself I'd make the best of it. Somehow, I did.

Six months after I'd taken the first Xanax, the psychiatrist told me to reduce the dosage by cutting the pills in half. I should take half a pill three times a day, he said, and come back in a month.

I downed the first half dose at bedtime and by morning, could tell I wasn't feeling quite as good as I had the day before. Shrugging my shoulders, I figured I'd tolerate it. I really wanted to reduce the dosage because I didn't want to become addicted to Xanax.

Not long afterwards, one morning while I cleaned house, I flipped on the radio. Before I got sick, I'd always had the radio on and sang while I cleaned. I stopped singing when I got sick, when it became an effort even to listen to the radio.

An announcer was talking about a preventive health clinic. It seemed like a message from God.

"If you are a woman having problems with menopause, depression, or hysteria, come in to see us."

I got on my knees. "Dear God, is this for me? Lord, what must I do? Will they be able to help me?"

I decided the next time I saw the psychiatrist, I'd ask how much longer I had to take the pills because I knew right then that the minute I got off them, if all the sickness came back, I'd go to the health clinic. It was my last resort. But until then, I'd trust the psychiatrist, stay on Xanax and Sinequan and give them a chance to work.

Just knowing I had another option, that I could go to the health clinic, made be feel better that day. It was good to know I hadn't yet reached the end of the rope.

Another month went by. During that time, I felt a bit more nervous in the morning, but nothing else was different.

When I next walked into the psychiatrist's office, the girl at the desk said, "Isn't it great to be talking to the psychiatrist? When I was really down, I saw him too. I felt so much better afterwards that I applied for this job and got it."

"I can't say I feel better," I thought, again wondering why I was there. Because my doctor ordered it!

After the psychiatrist called my name, I went into his office and tried to make myself comfortable in the huge leather chair. It wasn't easy. My clothes felt tight and I mentioned that I'd put on weight. "Is it because of the pills? My slacks are terribly tight and I feel bloated so much of the time."

Then I asked once again if I needed estrogen.

"Some people gain weight and others don't," he replied. "But you'll be on the medicine for only another month. As for estrogen, you don't need it."

One month to go! I was elated and forgot to mention estrogen again.

As he wrote out my prescriptions, the psychiatrist said I should again reduce the amount of Xanax I was taking and see how I felt. He said he'd see me next month.

At home as I cut the pill in quarters, I worried about how I'd feel with the lower dose. Would I get nervous again? The longer I thought about that possibility, the more frightened I got. I didn't want to get nervous and sick again, but I'd have to take that chance. I had to do what the psychiatrist said.

The next morning I felt more on edge than I'd been. "If it stays like this, I could tolerate it if I have to," I told myself.

A month later, I went for what I was hoping would be my last appointment. My head was reeling with questions. "Am I better than when I first came in? What will he say today? What happens when I stop taking the medicine?" But even though I worried about stopping Xanax, I worried even more about getting addicted to it.

To distract myself, I picked up a magazine and flipped through the pages. A lady sitting nearby started to talk. She immediately got my sympathy because she seemed extremely nervous. But when I realized that she wanted to talk about her family's problems, I got impatient and nervous myself.

"That's not why I'm here. I'm here only because the doctor said I needed a psychiatrist. It's been nine months now. I'll just have to be patient and see what God has in store for me."

I was relieved when the psychiatrist called me in. He was very nice and despite my misgivings about needing treatment, he did make me feel more comfortable. As I settled into the huge leather chair for the ninth time, he asked how I was doing.

"Ok," I replied knowing it would be stretching the truth to say I felt better. We talked for about ten minutes. Although he wrote another prescription for Xanax, he told me I should stop taking both the Xanax and Sinequan. "Get this filled only if it becomes absolutely necessary," he said.

"Will I get nervous again?" I knew he couldn't give me a definite answer, but I had to ask simply because I had such mixed feelings about whether I should go off the pills.

When we finished talking, the doctor shook my hand and wished me well. "If you need me again, remember I'm just a phone call away."

"Ok, doctor." On the way out, I paid the last bill and told the receptionist I didn't need another appointment. She seemed genuinely happy for me.

When Bob came home later that afternoon, as we got ready to go out for a Friday-night dinner, I told him the news.

"Good, I'm glad," he replied.

I wished I could be as happy as he was.

For the next ten days I woke up each morning feeling well but more than a little worried that it wouldn't last. But as each day progressed, I became more confident and I'd clean house, go shopping, visit a friend. Some of that confidence, no doubt, came from the "insurance policy" in my purse—the twenty-five pills that I'd gotten from the pharmacist, "just in case."

On the eleventh day, I felt weak and a little nervous so I took it easy and laid around all day. "I probably overdid it yesterday," I thought.

By the time Bob came home from work, I was really sick and when I told him, he got a very sad look on his face that said, "Not this all over again."

I went into our bedroom crying and stayed there all night even though I hardly slept. By the next morning I felt even worse and once again, suicide had crept back into my consciousness.

Bob left for work. I tried to force myself to think about anything but suicide, but it didn't work. With a heavy heart, I got on my knees and prayed. "How can I make it through another day, dear God? How long can I go on like this? Why are You doing this to me?"

Then I remembered the health clinic. "Should I call," I wondered. "Can they do something? Anything?"

I knew I'd try anything if it would keep me from going to a mental hospital. But if I called the clinic what would they tell me? Would they, too, say I had to go to a psychiatric hospital? Nothing had helped so far; how could they have anything that would make me feel better?

Underlying all my thoughts was the deeply embedded fear that I was so sick no one could help me. The mirror held the truth. A gaunt, old woman with a blotched face and no makeup; dark, sunken, lifeless eyes; quivering lips and limp stringy hair stared back at me.

I was frightened, but I had no choice. I couldn't give up. As long as there was somewhere to go, some new treatment to try, I'd find a way to get it.

"I'd better tell Bob." I dialed his number, but he wasn't there.

"Should I have him call you when he gets in?"

"Yes, please," I answered politely, suppressing the urge to demand that Bob call me immediately because I couldn't wait.

I paced nervously waiting for the phone to ring and hoping no one else would call first. I made some toast, but I couldn't eat it. At noon I debated whether I should go to the clinic without telling Bob, but before I made up my mind, the phone rang.

"I must go to a doctor, I must," I blurted out. "I can't stay here. I'm so sick."

Bob asked if I'd had lunch.

"No, I can't eat. I have to call the clinic. Can you eat lunch at home today?"

"I already had lunch."

I knew it was Bob's way of saying he couldn't come home. Of course not. How could I ask?

As always, Bob asked, "Will you be all right?"

"I don't know," I replied truthfully. "I just have to call them right now."

When we hung up, my hands were shaking so much that I could hardly dial the phone. I only knew I got the right number when a voice said, "Born Preventive Health Care Clinic."

7

The Long Road Back

January 26, 1988

I told the woman who answered the health clinic phone I needed to see a doctor right away, thinking, "I bet they never get calls like this, but so what if they think I'm desperate. I can't help it. Just please tell me I can come in before I do something terrible."

Before the woman replied, I added, "I'm extremely nervous and sick and weak. May I see a doctor?"

She sensed that it was urgent and checking the appointment schedule, asked if I could come in a little later that day.

What a relief, I thought, as I weakly replied, "Yes."

For three hours I watched the minute hand crawl around the clock and told myself to be patient. "What's three hours after feeling awful for three years?" As soon as the clock neared 3:30 p.m., I jumped into the car, drove to the clinic and walked through oversized glass doors into a waiting room dominated by a huge fieldstone fireplace and hearth. Unfortunately the room was filled with people who looked up as I entered. I didn't like having them watch me, so I found a seat in a somewhat isolated corner where they couldn't see how much I was trembling and waited to be called.

Finally a nurse called my name. She asked a few questions and when she finished, told me to go into the examining room and lie down. Within minutes, the doctor walked in. I'll never forget the compassionate, caring look on her face. I could tell she thought I looked awful and needed special care.

It was true. Considering the physical and mental state I was in, it was amazing I'd even made it to the clinic on my own. Only with God's help had I gotten there safely.

After hearing that I had had my ovaries removed surgically and listening to me talk about my symptoms, the doctor said, "You have an estrogen deficiency. I'm going to put you on estrogen right away. I'll give you a shot."

Instead of questioning her decision, I asked if I could take some Xanax to calm my nerves.

"Only if you really need it."

She explained that because of the severity of my symptoms I'd probably need another shot soon after the first and that I'd be able to judge when I should come in. We talked a while longer, then the doctor said she'd have the nurse come in to give me my shot.

"That's all?" I was surprised, but at the same time, pleased. I had come to the health clinic thinking I'd be sent to a psychiatric hospital and instead, I was getting a shot! And unlike the other doctors I'd visited, she hadn't said there was nothing she could do.

When the nurse came in with a syringe, she seemed sympathetic. "The doctor ordered an estrogen shot for you."

"Yes, something must be done," I replied, without elaborating. I was weary of repeating myself especially after so many doctors and nurses had made me feel like all my problems were in my head. "But God knows how I feel," I reminded myself. "He is the Great Physician, the Great Healer."

When the doctor came back, looking for more reassurance, I asked, "Doctor, will this help me?"

"It should help a little, but remember, you can come back for another shot in a week or two, as soon as you need it."

I relaxed in the examining room for about an hour after the shot until I felt calm enough to drive home. But once I got back in the car, I started crying anyway. Furtively dabbing my eyes—I didn't want anyone to see my tears—I prayed, "Dear God, Thou knowest how I feel. Could it be Thy will that this be the answer to what I am going through?"

At home I kept thinking of what I'd say to Bob about the clinic and the shot. I wanted him to know the shots might make me feel better, but still I hesitated. He hadn't said anything, but I knew he'd lost hope. He might not believe I had a chance to get well again and I, too, was struggling with doubt even though I desperately wanted to believe my doctor. On the other hand how could I keep my visit to myself, especially if it might be possible that all I needed was estrogen. Bob deserved a little encouragement, just as I did. We should both have some hope. So I sat impatiently at the kitchen table looking out the window so I'd see him drive up. And later when I spotted his truck, I couldn't wait for him to come in. I met him at the door and he heard every detail of my visit that afternoon.

For a week, I felt just a little more relaxed, but nothing else changed. I still felt sick and frequently thought about suicide. Then ten days after the shot, I could tell I needed more estrogen. I didn't know if they'd give me another shot so soon after the other, but I had to try. I felt desperate as I called the health clinic. I asked if I could talk to the nurse and when she got on the line, I explained that I'd had an estrogen shot ten days ago. "Can I come in for another?"

"Yes, you can," she said.

Breathing a sigh of relief, I asked when.

"Right away."

Hallelujah! God had answered my prayer again.

I didn't waste any time getting dressed and into the car. "The quicker I get there, the sooner I might get some relief," I told myself. I figured if the first shot helped, surely this one will help even more.

At the desk, I felt like a bundle of nerves. My legs were ready to buckle and my hands had a life of their own. They shook too much for me to hold a magazine, so I just waited to be called in.

When it was my turn, the nurse took my blood pressure, then asked me to follow her to an examining room where she'd give me the shot. As we walked down the hall, she explained that some women need more estrogen than others. "You are depleted, but should get a little relief from this shot fairly quickly," she said.

A little relief? Those three words told me my journey back to health would take time.

Later when I left the examining room, I met my doctor in the hallway. In her loving, friendly way, she asked if I had found any relief.

"Yes, somewhat."

"It will get better," she promised

"I hope and pray it will," I said, thinking to myself, "If I can come in often enough for a shot, maybe some day I'll be able to get on top of this."

In January, while I was still seeing the psychiatrist, Bob and I had made plans to go to our friends' condo in Florida the week of February 14. Bob wanted to relax in the sun for his vacation; I just worried whether I'd even be able to get there. The only reason I'd agreed to go was because the psychiatric medication I'd been taking for nine months had my nerves somewhat under control. Then two weeks after I'd stopped taking the Xanax and Sinequan, I felt like I'd been hit by a tank. All the symptoms came back so forcefully that what little estrogen I had gotten from the first shot was almost ineffective. I knew the second shot would not do much better, so Florida was out of the question. But what could I tell our friends? How could I say we couldn't go when they'd been so generous about giving us their condo for a week. They had other friends who would have jumped at the opportunity they'd given us. How could I say I was sick and nervous without sounding ungracious, especially since none of the other women in our circle of friends had ever suffered like this or even heard of anyone sick like I was. My excuses sounded lame, even to me.

"I hope they won't feel angry," I told Bob as I dialed the phone. As it turned out, our friends were very nice and only asked if we'd like to go in March or April instead.

"We'd like that. I'll let you know as soon as I feel better," I said.

I not only canceled Florida that month, but also another dental appointment and everything else on the calendar. We didn't invite anyone to our house and when friends called about going out for coffee, I'd say I wasn't feeling well. But I worried. If I kept giving the same old excuses, they might begin to think that I didn't want to be with them. I didn't need any more reasons for tears, but just the same, I now cried about what I thought our friends might be thinking!

I prayed that one day when I felt a little stronger, God would allow me to visit them. But it was difficult to believe I'd ever have any other kind of life. After so many months of wrestling with the same thoughts and prayers, I'd just about given up hope that I'd ever change.

A couple weeks after the canceled vacation and my second estrogen shot, I became even more desperate. I felt sick most of the time so I called the clinic and asked if I could come in again. The pleasant receptionist said she'd switch me to the nurse.

"God, please let them give me another shot," I prayed as I waited. "Even though there are times when I feel somewhat better and even though this is the best treatment I've had so far, I'm still very sick."

When the nurse came on the line, she said, "Yes, you may have another shot."

What welcome words. Now I had to figure out how I'd gather the strength to drive to the clinic. "Nonsense," I told myself. "I can't stay home. With God's guidance, I'll get there just fine."

The waiting room didn't seem quite as forbidding as it had on my first two visits. A small detail, but one that surely meant there was some small improvement in my health, I thought wryly.

Shortly after I sat down, the nurse called me in. "Are you getting some relief?," she asked.

"Yes, some." I wanted to ask how long it would be before I'd really feel better, but that question took more courage than I could muster at that moment. I knew I couldn't handle an answer I didn't want to hear.

Again, the nurse told me my estrogen was depleted.

Two injections and I still didn't have any estrogen in my system. I was hoping for a miraculous recovery so I could lead a normal life, but at that pace it would take months to feel well.

Adding to my despair was the knowledge that just a few days ago, on Sunday, I'd felt so awful that in desperation I'd called my physician again. When I asked him if there was anything he could give me, he'd responded somewhat sharply, "Just try to relax and don't worry about things. Take it easy!"

I'd fallen to pieces after talking to him. Then I prayed, "Dear Lord, when doctors can't do any more, will You do Your best work?" But I got no relief from my prayers that day. I had to let God take total control of my illness. Until He intervened, if it became absolutely necessary, I'd take Xanax. "But only under extreme circumstances," I promised myself.

Somehow I made it home safely after having my third shot. I tried to relax until Bob got home from work, then I told him where I'd been.

"Another shot?"

"Yes, I'm still very sick."

"I thought the last two helped."

"Yes, a little bit." I knew he thought I should feel much better but I didn't say anything.

The next few days were not good. Each morning I pleaded with Bob not to leave me alone. Then I had two days where it felt like the estrogen was working. I was a bit more relaxed, but not enough to go out or talk to friends or family. Talking seemed to increase my anxiety and sickness.

My body, which had been deprived of estrogen for eight years, was now at its lowest ebb. I was apathetic about everything, even how I looked. When friends told me, "You're losing weight," it didn't faze me.

I'd think, "I'm going to lose so much weight that I'll never recover."

By now, instead of trembling, my body quaked even while I was sitting or lying down. Stairs were a nightmare. I clutched railings so tightly my knuckles looked like snowcapped mountains.

But even though my future looked bleak, I never gave up my prayers and on those days when I felt too sick to pray, I had faith that God saw all my tears and knew how badly I was hurting. In the Book of Psalms 42, Verse 3, it says, "My tears have been my meat day and night while they continually say unto me, `Where is thy God?'"

I knew well the meaning of that verse. Each night I went to bed with tears in my eyes and when I woke up, I was crying. On sleepless nights, the tears slipped down my face relentlessly until morning.

March 9, 1988

Six days after my third shot, I knew I needed more estrogen, so I called the clinic again.

"Dear God, don't let them tell me that they can't do anything more for me." I lived with constant fear that if my doctor ever said there was nothing more she could do, I'd be in a psychiatric hospital for the rest of my life.

I asked the receptionist if I could see my doctor again and was overjoyed when she said I should come in that day. When I got there, I told the doctor I was still very nervous and sick. "Can something else be done? I'm desperate. I need relief. What I'm going through is terrible."

She said it was time for me to have an estrogen implant. "Do whatever needs to be done. I'm desperate and at your mercy," I told her. I didn't even ask what an implant was.

"I'll get my nurse in here and she'll explain the first steps."

After the doctor left, I started crying again. I was willing to try anything, but couldn't help worrying that the implant still wouldn't be enough to make me feel better. I was wiping tears when the nurse walked into the room a few minutes later. She explained the doctor would use a local anaesthetic to make a tiny incision, no more than a quarter-inch long, on my lower abdomen. Then the doctor would insert pellets of estrogen in the layers of fat between my skin and abdominal wall. Afterwards the incision would be closed with just one stitch and then I could go home. She said the doctor would be in shortly. Then while she scrubbed and sterilized a small patch on my abdomen, she started talking about the weather. I knew she wanted me to relax, but it didn't reduce my anxiety. Nevertheless, I appreciated her kindness and concern.

A few minutes later, the doctor came into the room. She showed me the small, three-piece metal instrument she'd be using to insert the estrogen between the fat layers. One piece looked a little like a hollow pencil with a pointed end that is worked between two planes of fat. Then she'd insert the estrogen pellets into the center piece, a short hollow tube that fits into the pointed "pencil." The last section looked a little like the pusher portion of a syringe. It pushes the pellets out of the center tube, down through the "pencil" and between the layers of fat. When the bottom section comes out, the pellets, about the size of saccharine pills, stay in the abdominal fat and slowly dissolve, giving off a constant supply of estrogen. When that supply runs low, my body will tell me, she said.

I liked my doctor and felt comfortable about the outpatient operation. She radiated sympathy, understanding and concern which meant a lot to me. I needed someone who listened and who understood what I was going through. Finally I'd found her, my new doctor.

"Do whatever you think best," I told her.

A few minutes later the pellets were in place. As she stitched the incision closed, she explained how I'd start feeling a little better just from having a constant source of estrogen. But any real improvements would take some time, she repeated. Then patting me on the shoulder, she assured me that eventually I would begin to feel like myself again. At that moment, I truly believed her.

"I'm going to have the nurse give you another estrogen shot before you go so you'll get some immediate relief," she said, adding, "If you have any problems, call me."

I left the doctor's office a short time later eager to tell Bob about the implant. When he got home from work, I told him my doctor was certain I'd eventually get well. But I could see he didn't believe me. He didn't say anything, but the expression on his face said, "What's next?" He simply didn't realize I was at the end of my rope and my only alternative was to try the implant.

The next few months were difficult. I had days when I could feel the estrogen taking hold—I felt more relaxed—but other days, it seemed to make no difference. There were times when I pleaded with Bob not to leave me home alone. I rarely left the house, not even for church, because I refused to go anywhere that I'd have to talk. Bob attended Sunday services and I watched them on TV, but if he knew I was too sick to be alone, then he'd stay home and watch them on TV with me.

Whenever friends came to the door or called on the phone, if Bob wasn't there to do the talking, I pretended I wasn't home. One evening as I lay on the sofa, the doorbell rang. I jumped off the couch and as I slipped into another room, I saw a friend at the door looking straight at me. I didn't care. I was willing to deliberately hurt her feelings and it gave me only a tiny twinge of guilt.

My friend was just one more in a long list of people I'd hurt in the last few years. By then, because of my reclusiveness a few of our friends had given up calling. I really didn't want to lose them and felt ashamed that I hadn't been able to prevent it. I prayed that some day I'd be able to explain everything and make it up to them. I wished this nightmare had never happened, but I knew God's ways are different than ours. He has a purpose and through my suffering, I was learning to put my life, my health and my faith in His hands. I thanked Him every day even though I still felt awful. Occasionally I had a sore throat or earache, but He had healed my allergies and asthma. And I no longer had to take the Xanax or

Sinequan. It was easy to find reasons to be thankful, especially when I knew He was still speaking to me.

August 15, 1988

Five months after my first implant, I knew I needed another. I decided to call the clinic, but before I did, I wanted to talk to Bob.

"In two months Rachel (our granddaughter) will have a birthday party. I want to go because if I don't, how will I ever explain to Jeff and Marianne why we didn't come. But the party's out of the question if I don't get more estrogen."

"You'd better call then," he answered.

Wondering what the doctor would say, I dialed the number and asked the nurse, "Can I come in for some more estrogen?"

She asked when I'd had my last implant and I thought, "Oh, no! She's going to tell me it's too soon. What will I do? I'll just have to take a tranquilizer!" I still had some left because even on days I felt desperate, I tried to use them sparingly.

"My last implant was five months ago."

Then she said the welcome words: "Come on in."

The next morning, I went to the clinic for my second implant. While the nurse prepped me, I told her I was still very nervous.

"It will take a while for you to feel right because your estrogen was depleted," she explained.

"Our granddaughter's having a birthday in a couple months. I sure hope I can go."

"You should be able to. It won't be long before you start feeling better and better."

"I hope so. I'd also like to wait a little longer than five months before I get the next implant."

When my doctor came in, she could tell the state I was in. "It will take time for you to feel a lot better," she cautioned.

I started to panic, but quickly calmed down. I could put up with waiting if I gradually improved. I'd just have to focus on knowing I was coming to the end of my suffering. Then it struck me that even though I'd been told it would take time before I got better, I had just received the best news I'd heard in years. Someday I actually would feel a lot better!

"Praise God, there is a cure for me!" I would just have to comfort myself with that message on my worst days, those days I despaired and thought I'd never improve.

After the surgery, the doctor again assured me that I'd eventually feel better. "But now," she added, "I'll give you another shot so you'll get some immediate relief."

Relief! What a joy that word was. On the way home, I thanked God that the clinic hadn't turned me away and that I'd had more estrogen. And naturally, the minute Bob walked in the door, I told him the good news.

The next morning I felt much more relaxed. Whether it was the estrogen working in my system or the message of hope I'd received, I don't know.

Four days after the second implant, I took out the stitch myself. That I could do such a thing had to be a sign I was indeed feeling better. I also went outdoors a couple times and told Bob I wanted to try going back to church.

On Sunday, even though I felt extremely nervous, I resolutely dressed myself. I had decided I'd go to church no matter what. I couldn't stay away forever and even if I did put it off for a week or two, I didn't think I'd be any less nervous than I was that day. Bob knew I was pushing myself because when I got in the car, my body started shaking.

"Are you going to be OK? Do you want to stay home?"

"I don't know if I can make it, but I'm going to try. If I stay home alone, I'll still be nervous. But let's try to sit in back so if I have to walk out, I can do it without everyone watching."

I knew God was beside me that morning and that His house would warmly embrace me. All I needed was a little extra strength. I asked Him to give it to me.

We were running a little late and when we got to the church, the parking lot was full of cars. That meant the church would be full too. I panicked. "Where are we going to sit? I don't want anyone looking at me," I told Bob. I knew everyone would notice us when we walked in and then they'd want to ask all kinds of questions. It was only natural that they'd wonder where I'd been, what was wrong with me, and why they hadn't seen me for such a long time. But I was in no condition to talk.

As we climbed the few steps to the sanctuary, I gripped the railing for dear life. At the entrance, I felt as though thousands of eyes were boring through me, so I loitered in the doorway refusing to be seated. If we sat down right away then people sitting nearby would still have time to ask questions before the service started. An usher asked if we'd like to sit in the fourth row, but Bob told him we'd rather sit in back. "Then you can get out easily if you feel worse," he whispered in my ear.

I don't know what the minister talked about that day. My lips quivered throughout the service and my eyes darted in every direction as I anxiously tried to spot whether anyone was watching me. I think the only reason I was able to sit through the whole service was because of God's loving concern. He had spared me a greater embarrassment, the embarrassment of leaving early and for that, I was thankful. As soon as service ended, we made our way back to the car. And I honestly don't remember whether anyone spoke to us that morning or if I so much as nodded my head in reply.

It was a relief to get back home. I felt good about what I'd accomplished, but that didn't ease what turned out to be a difficult day. I didn't eat anything because I felt nervous and sick, but I did manage to fix Bob's dinner. And I rejoiced that I'd finally gone to church. I knew the next time would be easier.

The two months between my second implant and Rachel's birthday slipped by. On one of my good days, I optimistically told my daughter-in-law Marianne that we would attend the party. Then on the bad days, I realized it would not be easy. No matter. Even if I felt bad, I was determined to attend. I owed it to Bob. He'd hate to miss one of the milestones in our young granddaughter's life.

Bob was in such great spirits the day of the party that I resolved not to say a word about how I felt. As it turned out, it was not one of my better days. I didn't say much at the party, but no one seemed to notice. We were together as a family again and for that blessing, we were all thankful. Watching my wonderful grandchildren play that afternoon was more of a thrill than I'd anticipated, especially since just a short time ago I had given up hope of ever seeing all my loved ones together again.

As we got up to leave, Marianne said, "I'm so glad you made it, Mom."

"I'm glad I did too."

I started crying when our grandchildren hugged and kissed us goodbye—tears of happiness! I slipped out the door before they noticed and got into the car. I still felt sick, but I was proud of myself for making it through the day. There are times when God gives us extra strength, usually when we need it the most, and for that, I thanked Him.

After that second implant, on days I could tell the estrogen was working, my symptoms just weren't quite as bad as they'd been and I'd feel much more relaxed. Then there would be days when I'd be so nervous it was even difficult to pray. But as it says in the Bible, (I Thes. 5:17) "Pray without ceasing." That was my guide.

By this stage, I found it somewhat easier to talk to Bob and members of my family, but I still had problems talking to friends and acquaintances. As a result, I continued to cancel appointments and change plans at the last minute.

The good signs were welcome, but I wanted more especially since our son Rick was getting married in a few months. There was no way I could stay home from his wedding, but I worried about all the relatives and friends who'd be there. "How will I be able to see them without talking? How will I ever get through the day?" I decided I'd just have to hide my nervousness and say no more than was absolutely necessary. I knew the wedding was going to be an endurance test, so I prayed that God would give me the strength I needed. But just in case I felt awful, I'd bring along some tranquilizers to back me up.

As it turned out, the wedding was not one of my good days, but I stayed at Bob's side all day long and thanked God that my husband didn't have to be there without me.

The wedding, nevertheless, marked a turning point in my life, a life that had been a shambles for so long. My good days were beginning to outnumber the bad ones. But because it was unpredictable from one day to the next, I still took each day one at a time.

Without Xanax and anti-depressants to improve my appetite, I was still losing weight. Food just didn't taste good so there were many days when I'd eat nothing at all.

I still didn't care how I looked. I threw on clothes which hung loosely from my bony shoulders. I washed my hair but never "fixed" it and I never bothered with makeup. My disheveled appearance gave me one more excuse to stay home.

Each morning I'd pray that God would give me the patience to get through the day. "Dear Lord, if it be Thy will, some day I will be totally healed. And if it is not Thy will, then please make my sickness bearable."

Some time after the wedding I started going out with Bob occasionally and sometimes I'd shop for groceries, always keeping one hand firmly attached to the cart because I still felt weak. When friends called, however, I usually refused to go anywhere even though I knew that the day was coming when I'd have to say yes. Bob very much wanted to be with our friends.

Finally one day to please him, I agreed to go for coffee, but I hardly spoke while we were out because my voice still quivered and I couldn't relax in a social setting. (Later it got so I could try to hide my nervousness instead of letting it overwhelm me.)

During this stage of recovery, I remember being outdoors one day when a neighbor came over to talk.

"Arlene, I think you are getting better. I could tell you were awfully nervous and you seemed so anxious. But now your voice sounds better."

"I'm not over it yet," I told her, "but I am getting better."

"Praise God," replied our wonderful Christian neighbor.

"You can say that again," I said, knowing that at that moment God was speaking to me through her.

Before my illness, I had taken not only my health, but also each day of my life for granted. Not anymore! I now savor the smallest blessings and thank God every day for people like my neighbor who has been such a wonderful comfort to me in good and bad years. On that day and many since, I felt much calmer just to be talking to her.

Although my life was improving by stages, full recovery was still a long way off. I wanted to visit family and friends, but accepted the fact that it was more than I could handle at the moment. I tried to attend church regularly, but sometimes the thought of having to say a word, even "hi" kept me home.

One day I met a young woman I'd known quite some time. She asked how I'd been and so I told her about my sickness and how I still hadn't completely recovered.

She said her mother had also become extremely nervous and unable to talk to anyone after a hysterectomy. Looking for answers, the family sent her to the Mayo Clinic, but it didn't help. The doctors couldn't find anything wrong with her.

"My mother came home," said the young woman, her voice breaking. "She later killed herself."

As the woman talked, a terribly sick feeling washed through my body, the same sensation I'd get whenever I heard the word "suicide" or an ambulance, whether it was outdoors or on TV. I'd get instantly nauseated and my heart would pound erratically like I was going to die.

I tried to say something to comfort my wretched friend, but I couldn't. I squeezed her arm and turned away trying to erase her words from my consciousness. How many times had I earnestly asked God to spare my life, I wondered. Now I knew with certainty that only through God's grace I had not committed suicide.

About six and a half months after the second implant, I could tell I needed more estrogen. When I told Bob and asked what I should do, he said, "There are days when you are feeling better. The estrogen must be working."

"Yes, it is." I didn't mention that I could tell I was getting better because the thought of committing suicide had almost disappeared!

"Call your doctor," he said.

I knew Bob couldn't let go of his fear that instead of improving, I'd get sick again like I had been before the estrogen treatments. He didn't want us to go through that again.

"I'm still sick," I assured him, "but not that sick. I'll be able to hold my own. But the clinic might say it's too soon for me to come in for more estrogen."

For a few days we debated about when I should call, but then I knew I couldn't wait any longer. So one morning before Bob left for work, I told him, "Here goes."

I knew the clinic's phone number by heart. I dialed, asked to speak to the nurse, and when she came to the phone, told her who I was.

"Oh, yes! What can I do for you?"

"It's been six and a half months since my last estrogen implant, May I have another?"

"I'll talk to the doctor," she said.

While I waited, I thought, "If she tells me "no," then the only thing I can do is bear it a little longer."

But when she returned, the nurse asked if I could come in the next day. My heart leaped at her welcome words and I replied, "Absolutely!"

Bob was delighted when I told him. "This time you should start feeling quite a bit better."

The next day when the doctor asked if I had noticed any improvements, I said, "There are times when I can feel the estrogen taking hold in my body. When I experience it working, it's great."

"You started taking estrogen a year ago and needed it very badly," she said. "With implants, pretty soon you'll be feeling great."

I wanted to believe her, but I still had bad days. "I do feel better sometimes, but it's been a long and trying year."

"I'll give you an estrogen shot right now and that should help," she said.

I always felt such joy in talking to my doctor. "You're a great doctor," I told her. "Don't ever let your mother get as sick as I did."

I knew the Lord was keeping me in His care. He had led me to my doctor, so I always thanked Him for sending me there. He had led me to the nutritionist too, and even though I always carried the old allergy and asthma medicine "just in case," I didn't need it. I simply didn't have allergies or asthma anymore. And whenever I wondered if I could make it through another day or night, I'd read Psalm 42:3 for comfort.

"My tears have been my meat day and night. While they continually say unto me, 'Where is thy God?'"

February 10, 1989

I no longer doubted that the source of my problems was my hysterectomy. Without ovaries to produce estrogen, I didn't have the hormone my body needed to function. As a result, I'd gotten allergies, asthma and everything else I'd had since 1985.

A few months after the third implant, my good days began to outweigh the bad ones. I started feeling well enough to go out with Bob more frequently and in addition, I no longer choked up every time I ate. That choked feeling had no doubt contributed to my nervousness. And by now I had enough experience to compare how awful I had felt taking tranquilizers and anti-depressants to the wonderful relaxed feeling I was getting from estrogen.

Despite my improvement, I still refused to go on a vacation or out of town overnight. I couldn't trust my body and if I felt sick, I wanted to be at home. It didn't bother me though. Feeling good was much more important than taking a vacation and "maybe some day I'll be able to go," I told myself.

As always I thanked God for how wonderful I felt. Ironically, sometimes I found myself crying while I prayed. These weren't tears of desperation, however, just tears of joy. They flowed as I repeated, "Thank you, Lord," over and over again.

Ever so slowly my life changed. I found myself answering the phone and talking to friends. I even initiated a few phone calls and on those days when I felt a little too nervous to talk, I just held off and called later when I felt better. We went out more often with friends. Even if I felt a little sick, I knew I could hide it because my vocal cords no longer quivered when I tried to talk. The other change I noted was that I no longer felt anxious. I was much more relaxed and went without worrying to several family parties. I also kept appointments instead of putting them off.

What a relief it was to start feeling normal again, but I often felt more pleased for Bob's sake than mine. I regretted how much he'd had to put up with and what he'd gone through. As long as I'd been sick, I can't remember hearing one complaint from him.

Then one day, for the first time in years, I really wanted to visit my mother and I wasn't at all worried about the 280-mile drive. So I called to tell her.

She was so happy. "Are you feeling a lot better?"

"Yes, there was a time when I didn't know if I would ever get to see you again, but now I have a lot of days when I am feeling a lot better. So we'd like to visit."

When I got off the phone, I started packing.

"Are you really able to do this," Bob asked.

"Yes, I think so. If I get sick, we'll just have to come home."

Throughout the drive, I felt very relaxed and prayed that it would continue so that we'd have a pleasant weekend. Shortly after we arrived, we suggested going out for dinner. We went to a nice little restaurant in town and I actually enjoyed the meal.

My mother kept telling me how well I looked.

"Yes, mother, I feel much better and food tastes good to me now so I'm eating better too."

"I'm so happy for you," she said. "You know, there were a lot of people praying for you."

"Mother, God is answering a lot of my prayers. Some of my symptoms are gone. I'm not nearly as weak as before and I no longer have to hang on to everything in case I fall. I feel more relaxed."

We had a wonderful evening and throughout the next day we talked and talked and shared a few joyful tears. It seemed as if we would never be able to make up for all the conversations we had lost.

On Sunday, my mother asked if I was able to go to church.

I gulped. It would be difficult. I had grown up in that congregation, so it made me more than a little nervous to think about going there. It was only natural people would want to talk to Bob and me.

I decided we'd go anyway, but I warned Bob he'd have to do most of the talking.

That morning I felt as though my nerves were being tested. But even though it seemed like a setback, I could feel the estrogen working and I knew that one day in the not-too-distant future, I'd be able to attend mother's church without a qualm.

August 23, 1989

Six and a half months after my third implant, I reached a point where I seemed to be getting just a bit more nervous. My bad days were nothing like what they'd been and I comforted myself with the thought that I was getting better all the time. Nevertheless I decided to ask if I could have another implant. "I'm not desperate," I assured myself, "but if they'll take me in, why not do it?"

When I told Bob what I'd decided, he quickly concurred. I knew he still had fears that I would get sick again and although I had reached the point of recovery where I felt better about myself—I even cared about how I looked—I, too, worried just a bit. Neither of us wanted to tip the delicate balance in the other direction.

I hoped they'd tell me to come in immediately, but knew I could accept it if they said I should wait a little longer. I called the doctor's office and the nurse asked if I could come in on Wednesday. Just two days away! "Sure," I told her happily.

I wanted to look good for that visit so I made an appointment to have my hair done and on Wednesday, put on some new makeup I'd just purchased. It was the first time I'd worn makeup in almost two years. I also put on a pretty blouse and earrings before driving to the doctor's office. I was early, but that was OK. I'd brought a book to read.

In the examining room a short while later while I waited for the nurse, I marveled at how much I'd changed. I wasn't all the way back to when I'd been healthy, but I definitely had come a long distance.

When the nurse walked in, she said, "Arlene, you look better!"

"I feel better," I replied. "I cannot believe how the estrogen can do all of this. It's a miracle!"

That day for the first time, I could tell the nurse how much I had suffered. She was sympathetic. Then the doctor walked in looking as beautiful as ever. Smiling, she asked how I was doing.

"Much better, doctor," I told her. "It's been a long time since I've felt so good."

"You look so much better," she replied.

Getting the same compliment from two people just a few minutes apart confirmed what I already knew. I also suspected that after this implant even more time would lapse before I returned for another implant.

"The implants are working just fine," I said.

Within months of the fourth implant, I realized I wanted to go out more and more frequently. It wasn't constant; on bad days, I still wanted to be home. But whenever I had a good day, I initiated an excursion to try to make up to Bob for all the times he had patiently stayed home with a sick wife. Even though he likes relaxing at home and working on his model trains and other hobbies, I knew there were times when I really pushed him to the limits of his endurance.

We began to babysit our grandchildren. We both enjoy them so much that all those months we had not had them over or done things with them had been very difficult for both of us. Their unlimited energy and motion no longer made me nervous or tired.

While I still felt short of breath, it was much easier to deal with it. My heart still thudded in my chest, but it wasn't the same heavy pounding that had made me fear I was having a heart attack.

And going to Sunday services was easier. I still avoided all the activities even though I was frequently asked to participate. I'd learned to say, "No," accept my limitations, and not worry about what people would think or say.

For the first time in three years, I truly was better.

I'd grown spiritually since 1985 and with real joy in my heart, I thanked God for each new day and for my new outlook on life, for bringing me so far and saving my life. He had answered all my prayers. I also thanked Him for leading me to the people who had a part in helping me get well.

My husband was astonished. He couldn't get over the difference in me. He, too, began to tell others what had happened and how I'd changed. He always says he will never forget what I went through. I won't either.

Jesus Took My Burden

Oftimes the way is dreary,
And rugged seems the road,
Oftimes I'm weak and weary,
When bent beneath some load;
But when I cry in weakness,
"How long, O Lord, how long?"
Then Jesus takes the burden,
And leaves me with a song.
I'll trust Him for the future,
He knoweth all the way,
For with his eye, He'll guide me
Along life's pilgrim way;
And I will tell in heaven,
While ages roll along,
How Jesus took my burden,
And left me with a song.
Yes, Jesus took my burden
I could no longer bear,
Yes, Jesus took my burden
In answer to my prayer;
My anxious fears subsided
My spirit was made strong,
For Jesus took my burden,
And left me with a song.

Rev. Johnson Oatman, Jr.

8

Recovery

March 1990

ABOUT two years after starting estrogen replacement therapy, I was functioning more like my genuine self. I was amazed that I could feel so well simply because I now had the vitamin and estrogen supplements my body needed to stay healthy. But despite the improvement, I still found myself thinking about everything that had happened in the last five years, and even more, how easily I could have been spared all that misery and heartache—and saved needlessly spent money. The old cliche was never more appropriate: "If only I'd known then what I know now."

I realized how necessary it is to take care of my body nutritionally.

Before I got sick, I'd always lived a fairly healthy life. I grew up in a strict Christian home which meant my parents never bought alcoholic beverages, not even beer. So as a child I didn't know what beer was or how it tasted. And as an adult, I followed my parents' temperate example. Whenever someone at a party or wedding would prod me to have a drink,

I'd say, "I don't drink." I don't care for milk and rarely drank soda either. I can remember my mother saying, "Water is like medicine" and her advice stayed with me. I usually drink as many as five glasses of water a day. In addition, I have to confess, I consume at least four cups of coffee a day. I can't give that up!

When I went to the allergist, the first thing he had asked was whether I smoked.

"No, never!" Smoking had never tempted me, not even the time in high school when I went out with two friends and one of them pulled out a pack of cigarettes and said we were going to have a good time. None of us smoked, but they were eager to try. They each took a cigarette and smoked it, then another. They kept begging me to take one, but I resisted and they eventually gave up. They really thought smoking demonstrated that they were grown up and glamorous and they couldn't wait to tell the kids at school. Later that evening, deciding they'd need proof, they'd asked me to snap their picture. I still have that photo of them in an old scrapbook, cigarettes in hand blowing out smoke.

A couple of years ago, when my sister and I were out together, we saw one of them and hardly recognized my old friend because her face was so wrinkled. Perhaps that came from her having smoked cigarettes most of her life. I gave thanks that day and many since, that I'd never gotten started and that I had taken the picture that day instead of being tempted to be in it.

Except for the years I went to one doctor after another, I've made a conscious effort to avoid taking pills, not even aspirin or Tylenol. People say Tylenol won't harm me, but I don't want any more medication in my body than I absolutely need. On those rare occasions when I get a headache—rare perhaps because I do not have any stress in my life—I take two extra Vitamin C tablets and drink six or more glasses of water instead of five, especially if I'm at home. If the headache persists, I just wait it out.

I don't take *Tums*—I've heard it can destroy the vitamins in your system—or *Pepto Bismal* or anything else to settle my stomach. And since street drugs weren't a problem when I grew up, they've never tempted me either as a youth or an adult.

I was raised on meat and potatoes and that's what my husband likes. He doesn't like frozen TV dinners, so most of the time, I've cooked "from scratch" using fresh or frozen vegetables and the better grades of meat, turkey and chicken. Our meals have always been very simple and plain, not spicy or greasy, but now more than ever we stay away from fried foods. We eat eggs, but not much sausage, ham or bacon. And when I'm making sandwiches, I use meat without fillers.

Because the nutritionist said wheat, corn, milk and rye are not good for people with allergies, I try to stay away from them. I never had a sweet tooth and now, with Bob having to watch his diet, we rarely have sweets or candy, particularly chocolate. I do buy some candy, cupcakes or cookies for our grandchildren, however, when I know they'll be at our house.

When we go out to eat, I like to order a bacon, lettuce and tomato sandwich on white toast. Very seldom do we get desserts in a restaurant; I just don't care that much for sweets.

Before I got sick, the only vitamins I'd ever taken were an occasional multi-vitamin. But after my respiratory problems, I started taking Vitamin A and zinc. Zinc is supposed to be good for women who have menstrual and menopausal problems and very little is found naturally in Michigan soil—and 500 mg. of Vitamin C several times a day. More recently I've also added Vitamin B6 Stress Complex, calcium and magnesium to the list. I'm very fussy about my vitamins; I always buy them at a health food store because I don't want to take any fillers or animal ingredients in my supplements. And since vitamins and minerals were all I had to lean on when I stopped taking allergy shots and asthma medication, and they've been very helpful, I never leave the house without them.

Over the last few years, I've tried to learn as much as I can about nutrition.

I like to listen to Herman Bailey's cable show from Florida. He often schedules guests who talk about nutrition. Whenever they're on, I stop whatever I'm doing, grab a pen and paper and take notes while I listen. That's how I started treating my headaches with Vitamin C and six or more glasses of water. One of his guests said it would work and although my headaches have never been bad or frequent, I find Vitamin C and extra water helps me too.

I've spent hours with the owner of the health food store. She's always there to listen and give advice. I've learned a lot over the years by talking to her informally and taking some of the nutrition classes she gives.

I've heard pros and cons about Vitamin C. Some people call it a miracle vitamin, others say it can poison your system if you take too much. I only know I've been healthier since I started taking 500 mg several times a day. Even my teeth seem stronger. Before I started Vitamin C and calcium with magnesium, I was always at the dentist (or canceling appointments when I was ill) for cavities, root canals, you name it. In 1985, I had nine fillings and three root canals; in 1986, three fillings and a bridge involving three teeth. I had one crown in 1987 and another in 1988, and in 1989, one filling and a crown. But since 1989, I haven't had one cavity. I go to the dentist three times a year for X-rays and to have my teeth cleaned and each visit, the dentist says they look good.

"It's because of my vitamins and calcium," I'll joke, not admitting how much I think it's true!

I don't have earaches anymore and rarely go to the doctor for antibiotics. If I do get a touch of a cold, it's brief. It's hard to believe that just a few years ago, when I couldn't breathe, I was sitting on the basement floor trying to catch my breath!

At one of my friend Pat Simmons' (owner of Pat's Health Food Store) nutrition classes, someone said a woman's periods can be heavy if she has an iron deficiency; now I wonder if that was what caused me to bleed so heavily before I had my hysterectomy. It was only because of the bleeding that my doctor recommended my surgery. Thinking back, I remember my mother had a similar problem. She had very heavy periods and a great deal of pain with her cycles, so when she was about fifty, she had a hysterectomy. I was in high school at the time. She always said she had a difficult time with her periods because of the hard work she had to do on the farm, picking stones, going up and down hills helping my father drag the land. Living on a farm was hard on women my mother's age.

Some time after her hysterectomy, when I was still in high school, I remember I was ironing in the kitchen. My mother sat in the breakfast nook cradling her head with both hands; they were on the table. I remember her saying, "Arlene, I think I'm going to die."

I was so scared, I didn't know what to do except to ask, "Mother, are you OK?" Sometimes she barely answered. Then the spell seemed to pass; she sat up and said she felt better. I remember they came over her a couple other times too, frequently enough that I finally mentioned it to my father. He said, "Mother doesn't feel very good at times." I also saw my mother crying a couple times, but I really wasn't home enough when I was in high school to say whether it happened frequently. I never found out why she had those spells; she never talked about it.

Other than that, my mother—and my grandmother, too—had long, active, healthy lives. They were both 86 when they died. And with their genes, except for

for those unfortunate years following my own hysterectomy, I hope I can expect the same.

At one time I took my good health for granted. Now each day is a special treat. I get plenty of sleep at night, try to lead a happy, Christian life and remember to thank God every day for His gifts.

9

I'm Not Alone

I often see my friend whose mother committed suicide. Her pain hasn't diminished; she still has trouble talking about it. She cries every time we meet, saying, "I wish I knew then what I know today."

She told me about all the doctors they'd taken her mother to and how no one could figure out what was wrong.

"My mother couldn't even talk to me. I wish she were here today."

"I understand. It's such a terrible sickness that when I was ill, I couldn't make anyone understand how sick I was. It's still difficult to explain today," I assured her.

One day I visited another friend I'd known for about three years. Before we knew each other she had been in a mental hospital twice with a severe case of nerves, but she had never mentioned it. Then I saw her again a couple days later and noticed how extremely nervous she was, but we didn't talk about it. A few days after that second visit, her husband called to say he had taken her to a mental hospital. So when I heard she was back home a few days later,

I stopped in for a quick visit. My friend still seemed quite nervous, but this time she talked about the hospital and all the different medications she was taking.

"When I was ill, I also took a lot of different medicine to calm me down," I told her.

My friend complained about ringing in her ears, so I mentioned all the earaches I'd had, as well as asthma and allergies. I told her I'd finally gone to a nutritionist and after I took the vitamins she gave me, my allergies and asthma cleared up. I also told her how the estrogen had helped me with my nervousness. "If it hadn't been for vitamins and estrogen, I would not be here talking to you today."

My friend seemed pleased that I'd talked about my problems and she kept asking questions. Then she said, "I'm going to see if I can take estrogen."

The next time I saw her, she seemed better. She told me about all the different tests she'd had and how her doctors couldn't find anything wrong. "But I'm much better," she added, "because now I'm wearing an estrogen patch."

That evening when my husband came home, I told him about my friend and what she had gone through. I mentioned that I knew about two other women with similar complaints.

"If I know three women, how many others are hurting too? I could have been spared all that grief if I'd known then what I know now. Women don't seem to be getting good advice. There's a need out there, Bob. Women should be informed and they should talk about this because it's such a terrible thing. I wish I could help them, and let them know they don't have to spend money on unnecessary drugs and all those different tests."

As I got stronger and healthier with each passing month, I frequently wondered how many women could be having problems like I'd had, especially those suffering from nervousness and unable to stop themselves from thinking about suicide. I wanted to help them, so I started asking God to show me the way.

Then one day I decided to put my experiences down on paper. Bob was startled when I told him because writing had never been easy for me. But once I sat down with a pen and paper, the words just flowed onto the pages. I quickly filled ten sheets. When I showed them to Bob, he smiled and said, "You wrote all of this already? I could never do that."

I kept writing and gave some of the pages to our children to read. Their overwhelming response was that I should keep going; they suggested that I should try to have the story published. I mulled it over. Then one day at the grocery store, I picked up a magazine that ran a health section and wrote down the address. I thought I'd send the editor what I'd written. But first it had to be typed. None of the family knows how to type, but my neighbor who has to do term papers was willing to help. When she finished, I sent the manuscript to the editors of the magazine and three or four weeks later got a reply. They politely told me they were unable to use my article and wished me success with another publisher. I went back to the store and got the address of another magazine with a health section in it. They, too, politely said no. That didn't deter me. My next letter went to *Prevention* and in four weeks they wrote back. By then, I was certain I'd have another rejection. To my surprise, they expressed interest and said they'd need my consent to publish. The story would appear when there was space in the magazine, they said. Some time later, they called, saying they needed a little more information, then my story would be published. It appeared in the November 1990 issue and afterwards, the response by phone and mail was overwhelming. Women called me to say that if we had changed the name in the article from mine to theirs, it would accurately describe their own experiences. One woman was in tears when she called, but after we'd talked for a while, she said she felt better. Another woman said she was happy to read it because it meant there was still hope for her. A third woman called my article "a life saver."

One woman sent a letter even though her hand wouldn't stop trembling as she wrote. As I read it, I relived so many nightmarish experiences so vividly that I started crying. The woman was desperate and wanted me to send any information I could get; she even wanted to know where I was going for my estrogen shots and implants.

Some women from a small town in Minnesota phoned and we talked for a long while. Afterwards, they went back to their own doctor who then got in touch with mine and my doctor generously shared her knowledge so that these women could be helped too. Now feeling better most of the time, the Minnesotans started a support group for women experiencing menopause and it reaches across state lines.

My circle of friends continued to grow as others heard about the *Prevention* article word-of-mouth.

I've been criticized for taking vitamins and estrogen and ridiculed for placing so much faith in what some people deem "quackery." But that's no reason I should stop telling my story. It isn't just about menopause. Women of all ages get hysterectomies and without estrogen, young mothers could be affected and that could compromise their ability to care for their children.

I can't tell any woman estrogen will work for her, just that it was the only thing that helped me. I want to let women know they should find out whether estrogen deficiency is causing their problems, that they have another possibility to consider when they are looking for answers.

My heavenly Father, the Great Physician, miraculously relieved me of my sickness. He gave me a wonderful husband who patiently struggled with me through all of this and who never complained about anything.

He led me to a doctor who lovingly took me into her care at a time when I had nowhere else to turn. She sympathetically saw my desperation and took time to talk to me and truly listen.

When I was ill, I didn't know why God had given me my burden, but I learned to trust Him. I've never questioned whether my story should be told or why God has selected me to tell it. So now if it is His will that I help others in His Name, I surely will. And to the critics, I say, "God has a reason for everything, all the things that happen in our lives. We are all on Earth for a purpose."

10

Bob's Story

I never thought Arlene needed a hysterectomy, but she wanted to follow her doctor's advice and in fact, he kept telling her she should have had the operation much sooner than she actually did.

After the surgery, our lives didn't change for a number of years. But then Arlene started complaining about allergies and they kept getting worse.

The first time I took her to the hospital, it was about 2 a.m. She had woken me up at midnight saying she couldn't get her breath. I told her to lie still and try to calm down and relax. But it kept getting worse, so we drove to the emergency room and stayed there while they ran some tests. The doctors didn't find anything wrong but they gave her something to make her quiet. On the way home she seemed better.

After that, Arlene started complaining about other problems. The second time we went to the hospital, the head nurse saw I was extremely upset. She implied I was being mean to Arlene and later, I got the third degree. I kept repeating that there was nothing like that going on, but I could tell the staff didn't believe me. I remember they had Arlene hooked up to a heart monitor and I kept watching it. Her heartbeat looked normal to me.

What I remember the most is how emotional Arlene became. She'd never been touchy before so it was difficult to watch her change.

No matter what I said, Arlene would get very upset and fly off the handle. There were times when she wanted me to leave the house. At other times, I knew she couldn't be home alone because she kept calling me at the railroad all the time just to talk or get some sympathetic relief. Then she started begging me to come home from work in the middle of the day. When I'd get home, she'd beg me to take her with me when I went back to work. I have to go out to repair railroad tracks and signals whenever I get an emergency call, so I told my boss Arlene was sick and we didn't know what was wrong. He let me take off whenever it was necessary and when Arlene didn't want me to leave her, I could take her along.

I was in a quandary all the time and often felt that no matter what I did, it would upset Arlene.

We couldn't go anywhere. Arlene wouldn't talk to anyone, not even our own children. She wouldn't go to church and I always had to answer the phone. I remember the time her mother called and I had to tell her gently, in the best way I could, that Arlene couldn't talk on the phone.

We didn't have much of a life during those years. I consider myself a patient person and realized I had to make the best of it. Nevertheless, it was a depressing time for both of us.

When I'd come in from work, I never knew what to expect. I didn't know if Arlene would be crying or if she'd just want me to leave. She was very emotional and anxious, with terrible mood swings. If I said one word the wrong way or in the wrong tone of voice, she'd get upset and start to cry. At one point, she even said, "Just go away," because she was so nervous.

When the doctors said there was nothing more they could do for Arlene, I really started wondering if I would have to commit her to a mental institution. I couldn't shake the thought that she'd end up in a hospital. If the doctors couldn't do anything more, undoubtedly she'd end up there and I would have to accept it. I couldn't help wondering if I was going to spend the rest of my life alone.

I was skeptical when Arlene said she wanted to go to the Born Clinic but I knew no matter what I said, she'd do what she wanted. I felt we were clutching at straws, but anything was better than the alternative, a mental ward.

After she started on estrogen, there was a gradual improvement and after a while, even I began to harbor some hope. It was an emotion I'd not had in a long time.

Now when Arlene talks to women about how serious it is to have a complete hysterectomy and what can happen afterwards if they don't get the estrogen replaced, I tell them she is telling the truth and talk about how terrible our lives were at the time. I warn them that if they don't get enough estrogen, it could have a devastating effect on their bodies and minds.

I can't help but place blame on the doctors who were unable to diagnose the cause of Arlene's illness. They, of all people, should have known the body is a complex mechanism and for that reason, she should have been placed on estrogen immediately after her surgery to counteract any damage or imbalance that might occur with having the ovaries removed.

I think we need to educate women about the devastating effects a hysterectomy can have when estrogen is not replaced.

11

The Professional Perspective

WHY don't women know more about estrogen? Why do some doctors put women on estrogen replacement therapy while others don't? And why are so many patients in their change of life sent to psychiatrists, and given tranquilizers and anti-depressants instead of hormones?

Most of the research conducted has been geared towards men so little is known about menopause and estrogen. Research for women's health has not received much funding, especially because for a long time it was assumed that any studies focusing on men would also apply to women.

In addition, the medical community, primarily male, has not been interested in menopause or treating menopausal patients. So when a woman comes in with vague complaints, doctors may not actually listen to what the patient is saying. And when the various tests come back "normal," these doctors may attribute the patient's complaints to emotional stress brought on by external factors that cause stress in a woman's life. Doctors also tend to rely on oral estrogen to treat patients and when the pills don't work, they decide estrogen isn't causing the patient's problems.

Complicating the picture is the controversy about estrogen and cancer. Some studies suggest estrogen increases the risk for women getting cancer especially if they take it for a long time. Other studies indicate that use of estrogen by menopausal women actually helps them prevent heart disease and osteoporosis, the loss of calcium which leads to brittle bones in aging women. So much of the debate centers on the pros and cons of long-term use of estrogen.

Women themselves don't know much about menopause. It rarely was discussed by female members of their families and women rarely talk about it with friends, unless they're having problems and looking for the reason why they feel as they do.

For thirty years Tammy Geurkink, D.O. and her husband Grant Born, D.O. have helped hundreds of women searching for help with menopausal symptoms. They specialize in estrogen replacement therapy at the Born Preventive Health Care Clinic and have been giving estrogen implants to patients since the late 1960s when Dr. Born was licensed by the federal Food and Drug Administration to clinically test and document the effects of the then experimental drug. The FDA eventually authorized implants for general use based on the data submitted each month by Dr. Born and roughly one hundred doctors nationwide. All experimental drugs have to go through a similar process with the FDA.

So what is menopause and when does it start?

For most women the early signs of menopause (perimenopause) occur when they approach fifty and roughly seven to ten years later, when they've not had a menstrual cycle for a year, they actually reach menopause (the end of menstruation). For most women it is a "natural" process, meaning they generally experience a gradual reduction of hormones and their bodies have time to adapt to the fluctuating and decreasing levels of estrogen. Therefore, for most of them, the various symptoms they experience are, for the most part, manageable.

Another group of women also experience menopause naturally, but they start having symptoms when they are in their late thirties or early forties. (According to an August 1994 survey in *Prevention,* a larger group of women in their early forties reported they were perimenopausal than was expected. But the majority of women said they were about forty-eight when they started having symptoms.) Some women may be even younger than thirty-seven or thirty-eight when they start having symptoms of menopause. It happens when their estrogen level does not bounce back to normal after they have delivered a baby. Because this group of women is "too young" to experience the symptoms of menopause, they may not get treated when they go to the doctor for help.

"People have preconceived notions about who's supposed to be in menopause, but it's not strictly women in their fifties who are having problems," says Dr. Geurkink, recalling a patient who was in her early thirties with an estrogen level of two. Another was a woman in her mid-thirties who complained of living with "a pressure," as well as headaches and other symptoms. With one shot of estrogen, the patient felt fifty percent better.

"Women whose bodies are not cooperating know what their lives used to be, how they used to feel and how well they used to sleep. After a while, low estrogen magnifies those changes and suddenly the mountain is unattainable, it becomes a formidable object."

Dr. Geurkink's opinion is supported by Lonnie Barbach in her book, *The Pause, Positive Approaches to Menopause*. "Many physicians simply do not understand the transition to menopause is a process that can take years. A woman can start as soon as the late thirties or early forties—from two to ten years before her last menstrual period and a year or so after."[1]

Almost one third of the women in menopause have had hysterectomies. About fifty percent of them were subject to becoming depressed and having problems that could occur as much as two years after the operation, according to an article about menopause that appeared in the *San Modesto Bee*, California.[2]

It does not make any difference whether or not they still have an ovary!

When the ovaries are removed, women are going to have problems no matter what age they are, says Dr. Geurkink. Even if they have one ovary, it becomes ineffective and usually within a year, most of these women will become menopausal. But even while that one ovary is functioning, most women don't feel good because one ovary simply cannot produce what two did. It leaves them with less estrogen than they used to have.

The hysterectomy itself may cause changes that cause the ovaries to shrivel up. During surgery, some of the blood supply to the ovaries is cut. So even though the main major arteries are left in tact, the ovaries don't work as well as they did. "They know they don't have a reason to produce as much estrogen and they get slower. Whether it's because of blood changes resulting from surgery or the stresses of the surgery, no one knows why."

What are the signs of menopause?

One of the first symptoms that women experience is insomnia. Second is a mood change; women become more irritable and teary. Along with that their periods may become irregular-they'll either start too quickly after the last period or their periods may be heavier than normal. Further down the scale, women usually start getting heat intolerance, anything from warm flushes to feeling warm all the time to waking up with night sweats. Almost always, they are fatigued and the little things women used to be able to handle, like a schedule, become overwhelming. They may wake up in the middle of the night. They may have a lowered sex drive or pain during intercourse and they may become forgetful. In severe cases, women may become depressed and experience anxiety, panic attacks and palpitations (the "quaking and pounding heart" described earlier in this book).

Approximately ten-to-fifteen percent of the women going through menopause experience severe emotional and physical distress. (The percentage could be somewhat higher, according to the survey published in Prevention. The magazine reported that twenty-six percent of the two thousand readers, randomly selected from a response of fifteen thousand, reported that they had experienced bouts of anxiety and depression. None of the women included in the study had had a hysterectomy.) According to statistics, fifteen percent of women in menopause say they have no problems and about seventy percent report some symptoms, but for the most part they are manageable.

In her book, *Estrogen: Is It Right for You?,* Paula Dranov said, "After a hysterectomy, the sudden loss of estrogen brings on symptoms usually much more severe than those that occur when menopause arrives naturally, following a long and gradual decline in estrogen levels."[3]

And in *Transformation through Menopause,* Marian Van Eyk McCain, said when the ovaries are gone, a woman "no longer feels she is inhabiting the same body-she might even begin to wonder who she is.[4]

What happens when those women visit their doctors?

They might not get treated if their doctor relies on the results of estrogen level tests. If the level is in the normal range—anywhere from five to 375 micrograms—the doctor will say the patient doesn't need estrogen. But "normal" lab values aren't always an accurate measure of whether a woman needs estrogen, says Dr. Geurkink. "You may get a level of one hundred and it's within normal limits. But if a woman is used to having three hundred micrograms, she's only getting one-third of the estrogen she used to have. The estrogen level is simply not the right way to look at it."

Also, there are doctors who believe women must be almost fifty before they can become menopausal. Other doctors believe women should not be treated with estrogen until after they have stopped menstruating for a year. Add that to the group of doctors who do not listen to what their patients are saying and the likely result is a sizeable group of women who may not be getting estrogen to relieve their symptoms.

Most of the women who come to Dr. Geurkink have been taking estrogen, but they are still having problems. That happens when the method of administering the estrogen is not correct or when they are not given the right balance of estrogen and progesterone.

Doctors generally prescribe hormones taken orally and if the pills don't help, they'll tell their patients they don't have an estrogen problem, says Dr. Geurkink.

Why doesn't the pill help?

The pill works best for women going through menopause naturally, but even within that group, some won't get enough estrogen from the pill. Because it is taken orally, it has to go through the digestive system and that means all the right digestive enzymes have to be present to absorb it. After it has gone through all the stages of absorption and through the liver, whatever estrogen the liver has not metabolized works through the system. And that's what's left for "functional" estrogen.

The patch delivers estrogen more effectively because it bypasses the digestive system. Placed directly on the surface of either the abdomen or buttocks and changed every three and a half days, the estrogen on the patch is absorbed through the skin. "The one or two milligram dose delivered over a three-day period works best for women who are already into menopause and are used to having low levels of estrogen, but it is not a lot of estrogen for most young women," says Dr. Geurkink. They would do much better with injections of estrogen. Depending on their general health, their age, and how much stress they're under, a shot can last anywhere from a week to six weeks. Most women get a shot every two-to-four weeks.

The implant which releases a steadier, more even level of estrogen as it dissolves is best for women who have had hysterectomies and those who get a roller coaster effect from shots. Implants generally last about six months. But in cases where a woman's body has been totally deprived of estrogen over a long period, estrogen from the first few implants and supplementary shots may be depleted very quickly. "No one knows exactly why," says Dr. Geurkink, but it may be that the estrogen gets metabolized quicker or until the deficits that occur when the body is deprived of estrogen are filled. (Estrogen is often stored in a woman's fat cells.) Eventually, when her system reaches an equilibrium or a balance between the available hormones and the woman's lifestyle, the implants will last longer.

Why don't women know more about menopause?

They don't learn much from their mothers and rarely discuss it with their doctors or their friends, at least not until they start having problems. After all how many women want to draw attention to the fact that they're aging, especially when they live in a society that worships youthful women with beautiful, thin, bodies. Middle-aged women are not regarded as having sex appeal and they are not valued for their experience and knowledge. Instead they're stuck with unflattering stereotypes. So the last thing any woman wants to do is draw attention to the fact that she's in menopause.

In an excerpt from her book *The Silent Passage: Menopause,* Gail Sheehy attributed the "silence and apprehension" about menopause to phobias about aging-young women are considered desirable, older women do not have well-defined roles, and women allow themselves to become victims of menopause by becoming inactive, getting fat and losing interest in sex. "They perpetuate the stereotype of the menopausal woman as a mean, old bitch."[5]

"Midlife women have been faced with not only sexist but also ageist attitudes, which discount and dismiss the very real concerns of menopausal women.

Rather than label ourselves as 'menopausal' and thereby invite the negative stereotype of the middle-aged complainer, too many of us have kept silent," said Janine O'Leary Cobb in her book *Understanding Menopause.*[6]

Our society judges women by their beauty, clothes, figures and youth. If that's the basis for their self-esteem and the way they've always attracted men, when they become middle-aged, they often don't value themselves, said Dr. Sadja Greenwood in her book *Updated Menopause, Naturally.*[7]

As a result, women may enter midlife expecting to have hot flashes and they may know their monthly cycles will eventually end, but little else. And when they seek help for intolerable symptoms of menopause, that's when they realize doctors don't have answers.

Until recently medical studies on women's health received only one percent of the research funding allocated by the federal government. The other ninety-nine percent went towards research about men.

"If men had their testicles surgically removed when they are in their thirties and forties," says Dr. Geurkink, "you can be sure we'd know a lot more about testosterone than we know about estrogen and menopause."

"Social customs, health policies and a largely male medical community have tended to treat women as wives or wombs and little else. Consequently, as chronicled in report after report, aspects of women's health, including nutrition and aging . . .

have received minimal attention or funding. Gaps pockmark the formal knowledge of women's health," said Marguerite Holloway in an article in *Scientific American.*[8]

In an article in *Health,* Amanda Spake confirmed that opinion. "The kinds of studies that could pin down the benefits and risks of various types of hormone therapy—well-controlled clinical trials—simply haven't been done."[9]

As Dr. John Arpels pointed out in Lonnie Barbach's book *The Pause: Positive Approaches to Menopause,* men represent 49 percent of the population and dominate the ivory towers of medicine and "until recently women have not been taken seriously enough to generate the necessary studies."[10]

"The important events in a woman's life (menstruation, pregnancy, childbirth and menopause) have never been taken very seriously by the male political or medical establishments," said Janine O'Leary Cobb in *Understanding Menopause.*[11]

Happily, the pendulum is swinging. Women are becoming recognized for their unique health concerns and thus are the focus of several important new studies currently under way. The recent emphasis on women might have been helped by the fact that more of the people conducting research are women, a growing group of doctors are female and want answers to their patients' problems, and a large group of baby boomers are very likely experiencing perimenopause themselves. But even though the studies are underway, the results won't be available for years.

Why do some women have problems with menopause?

It should not come as a surprise that there's little agreement on why some women suffer severe emotional and physical distress, whether low estrogen levels contribute to the problem and whether estrogen replacement therapy actually helps or should be avoided.

Women themselves can't agree whether they should take estrogen or if instead, they themselves are responsible for determining methods to treat symptoms, says R. Margaret Voss, Ph.D., a Grand Rapids psychotherapist who has led group sessions on menopause for the last four years. Group discussions "have been valuable because they help eliminate women's fears. Women learn they are not alone in their symptoms and they're not crazy. And in group we help them formulate questions to ask their doctors."

When ten to fifteen percent of the women in menopause start having extreme physical and emotional reactions, their problems are likely to be attributed to depression caused by external factors that occur at the same time of life as menopause: mid-life changes experienced by husbands that may lead to divorce, the normal struggles of parenting teens, the empty nest syndrome, aging parents who may need care, and the unexpected and sometimes traumatic job changes—buyouts, transfers, or losses.

If doctors attribute the problems to anything but a woman's physical health, no wonder some of them still use quick, easy and traditional ways to treat their patients: tranquilizers and anti-depressants. These powerful drugs are prescribed to keep women quiet and if they don't work, women may be sent to a mental hospital.

Too often women's problems are regarded as emotional, says Dr. Geurkink. Many of her new patients come in carrying thick folders filled with medical records. Some of them have just been released from a psychiatric hospital. "They're not all fearing they will commit suicide, but their lives are being seriously impacted by estrogen deficiency."

Dr. John Arpels, founder of the North American Menopause Society, agreed. In Lonnie Barbach's book *The Pause,* he says too many of his patients have "had to be taken off Prozac, prescribed by internists for mid-life crises, when their problems actually were caused by the estrogen phenomenon. Most physicians just don't understand this at all."[12]

"Menopausal women with physical or psychological problems are frequently given potent medication instead of the information and counseling they may need," said Dr. Greenwood.[13]

And O'Leary Cobb, who publishes *A Friend Indeed,* a newsletter for menopausal women in addition to writing books, says doctors "are often ill equipped to handle a discussion of mood swings, anxiety, panic attacks and depression. When they refer patients to a psychologist or psychiatrist, the patient feels that her problem is being redefined as emotional or mental, when she feels, and often rightly, that it is the result of stress on the body."[14]

After the article in *Prevention* appeared, Dr. Geurkink received a call from a Wisconsin lawyer who wanted more information about estrogen deficiency. He had a client who had just been released from a mental institution. Committed by her family, the woman had been taken to the hospital in a strait-jacket. She spent two years in the hospital before learning that her emotional instability was the effect of estrogen deficiency. After she was finally released, she wanted to sue the hospital, her doctors and her family for the two years of her life that she'd lost.

What can doctors do to avoid a misdiagnosis?

"Listen," says Dr. Geurkink. "It's very important to listen. Most of the time a patient can tell a doctor what's wrong if the doctor is listening objectively. But all doctors come with preconceived notions about who should be in menopause."

How does Dr. Geurkink determine which patients need estrogen? "Most people who seek treatment at the clinic aren't being helped by their hormones. I take estrogen levels to monitor a person's progress, but don't use it as a total diagnosis. I go by how a woman's feeling, whether she's depressed, not sleeping, having periods every six weeks and is fatigued. I'll give her a shot of estrogen and if she's feeling better on injectable estrogen, usually within twenty-four hours—and with some women within twenty minutes—you can pretty much be assured that the estrogen she's getting from the patch or pill is not effective. That first shot won't do any harm, but it won't last long because of the estrogen deficit.

"Before you give any more estrogen, you have to make sure the patient doesn't have cancer because estrogen does make an existing cancer worse. I give a physical exam and use the mammogram, PAP smear and a colposcopy to detect early cancers. In addition, every time a patient on estrogen comes in for an office visit, she gets a free colposcopy to check for atrophic changes such as thinning of the vaginal wall." Dr. Geurkink uses the colposcopy to monitor patients on estrogen for cancer because PAP smears are only fifty percent effective.

Most of the debate about estrogen replacement therapy centers on two questions: Does a woman risk getting cancer if she takes estrogen? And does that risk increase if it is taken over a long term? Although estrogen is known to accelerate growth of an existing cancer, there's no concensus about anything else. But since some studies suggest a woman's risk for cancer increase if she takes estrogen for a long time, some doctors will not prescribe estrogen and some women refuse to take it.

Winifred Gallagher said in the *Atlantic Monthly,* "In evaluating the effect of hormone replacement therapy on physical health, women and doctors must juggle evidence suggesting that while HURT cuts the number of hot flashes by about half and reduces vulnerability to osteoporosis and perhaps coronary disease, it may raise the risk of breast cancer and, if estrogen is taken without progestin, uterine cancer." One group of doctors lets women make their own decision; others recommend hormone replacement therapy only for those whose risk of breast cancer is low, while a third group "regards the use of hormone replacement therapy with dismay."[15]

Karen Steinberg, a molecular biologist at the Centers for Disease Control and Prevention, quoted in an article in *Health* said the risk of getting cancer is small. An average woman has a ten percent chance of developing breast cancer some time in her life and if she takes estrogen for fifteen years, she might increase that risk to thirteen percent. And in the same article, Malcolm Pike, a University of Southern California epidemiologist, said for each additional breast cancer death caused by taking hormones, eight deaths from heart disease can be prevented. "We already know that hormone replacement therapy is beneficial to the heart, it's very good for your bones, it makes you feel better—but it may give you cancer. Still, if you want to live long, you take it."[16]

"There's no single right, risk-free answer. Every time you put something in your body you take a risk. You also take a risk when you do nothing and perhaps, you're depriving your body of what it needs," said Lonnie Barbach in *The Pause.*[17]

"There's a lot of bad press about estrogen," says Dr. Geurkink. "I don't think it's been shown it can cause cancer, but if cancer's already present in a woman's system, yes, you can make it worse by taking estrogen. High levels of estrogen unopposed by progesterone may influence development of endometrial cancer. But it's the immune system—the overall ability the body has to handle cancer—that determines why some women get cancer and others don't.

"The immune system needs antioxidants to help it along. Oxidative stresses cause damage, much like oxidation causes rust on metals, so we have to be careful about keeping the antioxidants elevated.

"There are things a patient can do on her own to balance any effect estrogen may have negatively to stimulate cancer," she adds. "We can elevate a patient's antioxidant status if she takes Vitamin A, Vitamin E which is extremely important, Vitamin C, beta carotene and glutathione, which helps the liver detoxify certain toxins since the liver is capable of handling only a limited level of toxins each day. The dosages of each vitamin vary from patient to patient." Some foods, herbs and teas also elevate the antioxidant level.

Another way to diminish possible risks of cancer is to reduce the amount of estrogen taken. Some of the other methods of administering estrogen will give most women less estrogen overall than they'd get from the pills.

A daily dose of the pill Estrace, usually one or two milligrams, adds up to thirty or sixty milligrams of estrogen a month. In addition, the patient gets the fillers, chemicals and food colorings pharmaceutical companies use in manufacturing the pills.

A shot of estrogen, however, gives a woman only two-and-a-half to five milligrams of Estradiol, Estrone or Estriol. And since most women only need one or two shots a month, their actual estrogen intake is usually no more than ten milligrams of estrogen a month.

Pellets reduce the total intake of estrogen even more because a twenty-five to fifty milligram dose typically lasts six months or longer.

Throughout history most women went through menopause without needing supplementary estrogen. What has changed?

Two possibilities stand out. Women have longer lifespans than their mothers and grandmothers did and in many ways, they are much more active. Women's lifestyles have changed. They have careers in addition to their families and they experience more stress from busy schedules. And when they delay pregnancy until they are in their thirties and occasionally, forties, that means they'll have young children and teen-agers at home when they become menopausal.

"Some women will do fine with low hormones, but a lot are going to need estrogen well past the time of menopause because of these lifestyle changes," says Dr. Geurkink. "You have to judge each person individually. But if it doesn't do a woman any harm, why not let her live a healthier, happier life. Estrogen is anti-aging. It keeps your bones healthy. It keeps your arteries healthy, your skin strong and your cholesterol and triglycerides down. There's probably no reason to go forever without hormones."

References

1 Barbach, Lonnie, Ph.D., *The Pause: Positive Approaches to Menopause,* A Dutton Book, New York:1993, p.7.

2 *Hysterectomy Toll Underestimated,* Health & Science M.D., Modesto Bee, California: Nov. 8, 1988.

3 Dranov, Paula, *Estrogen: Is It Right for You?* Simon & Schuster, New York: 1993, p.13.

4 Van Eyk McCain, Marian, *Transformation through Menopause,* Bergin & Garvey, New York: 1991, pp.28-29.

5 Sheehy, Gail, *The Silent Passage: Menopause,* Vanity Fair, October, 1991, p.252.

6 O'Leary-Cobb, Janine, *Understanding Menopause,* Toronto: Key Porter Book, 1988, p.5.

7 Greenwood, M.D., Sadja, *Updated Menopause, Naturally,* California: Volcano Press, 1992, p.82.

8 Holloway, Marguerite, *Trends in Women's Health: A Global View,* Scientific American, August 1994, p.77.

9 Spake, Amanda, The Estrogen Question: *The Raging Hormone Debate,* Health, January/February 1994, p.48.

10 Barbach, L., p.xiii.

11 O'Leary-Cobb, J., p.5.

12 Barbach, L., p.37.

13 Greenwood, S., p.86.

14 O'Leary-Cobb, J., p.52.

15 Gallagher, Winifred, *Midlife Myths,* The Atlantic Monthly, May 1993, pp.55-56.

16 Spake, A., p.50.

17 Barbach, L., p.10.

12

Epilogue

January 1995

I'VE now had eight implants and will soon get my ninth. They usually last about six or seven months. Then I start feeling a little weak and my back might hurt a little; they're my "signals" that it's time to go back to the clinic.

The implants work best for me. I tried estrogen patches for about a year while implants weren't available, but they didn't deliver as much estrogen as I need to feel well. Luckily I'd already had four implants, so my body wasn't totally depleted of estrogen when I switched to patches. Otherwise I think some of my symptoms might have gotten pretty bad again.

A patch lasts about three and a half days, then you place a new one on your skin (usually the buttocks or abdomen). The estrogen on the patch is like a gel and is absorbed through the skin into your blood stream. Women who have not had hysterectomies may get enough estrogen from the patch. But women like me, who have had their ovaries removed, get a much steadier supply of concentrated estrogen from the implant. I seem to need every ounce of estrogen I can get.

My recovery did not come quickly. It was at least two years before I felt more like my old self. But it's no wonder it took so long to build myself back up. I'd gone without estrogen for seven years before starting replacement therapy.

Even with the implants, there are times when the natural ebb and flow of life robs me of estrogen. I noticed it particularly when my mother died three years ago. She had been in a hospital for five months before passing on and the stress taxed my nerves and my estrogen as well, just as it would have done with any other woman. But I'm pleased to say I handled those horrible months without suffering a relapse.

Now I can truly say I feel as good as I did before my hysterectomy. My life is back to normal. I don't have any aches or pains. Other than my vitamins, minerals, and estrogen, I don't need to take any medicine. And best of all, they are not drugs; they are natural ingredients that belong in my body.

I lead a very busy, active life. Bob and I get up at 6:45 a.m. and don't stop until 10 or 10:30 p.m. (I never nap!) I've always enjoyed housework and cheerfully plunge into cleaning, laundry and all the other chores that never seem to end. But my favorite activities are gardening and taking care of our grandchildren. I'll work all day in my flower garden and then willingly spend the evening caring for one family of kids or another. We have eight grandchildren now and another is on the way. Two of them live across the street from us. The minute the Michigan climate warms up, if they can't find me in the house, they know to head for the yard. There they'll help me weed, plant and fertilize flowers all summer long. They're actually becoming good little gardeners themselves.

When we go up north for a weekend to my mother's old home, which we purchased after she died and are fixing up, a lot of times Bob and I take a couple grandchildren along. They're always eager to have their turn because they enjoy having some special time with us. Some day we'd like to go on a vacation with all of them at once, as well as our sons and their wives.

I think my time with our grandchildren is especially precious because of what I went through. I cherish that time together and am thankful that I had the illness when I did. Because at that time the two oldest grandchildren were too young to notice that I wasn't involved in their lives. Now, without having to worry about my health, I enjoy each one of them and the particular stage of development he or she is going through.

I like quiet time too. I've always been fairly self-sufficient and slightly reserved; it comes from growing up on a farm and having only one sister for companionship. We lived far enough from town (where most of our classmates lived) and had so many chores to do that we rarely took part in our classmates' social life or extracurricular activities at school. So it was only natural, especially as we got older, that we really weren't part of the crowd. After high school I worked at a local hospital with two classmates. The three of us rented two bedrooms on the second floor of a house in town. Even then I was on my own. My classmates shared one room and I had the other so I still tended to keep to myself. It didn't matter, because I've always enjoyed reading. I like to read all the literature and mail put out by "Concerned Women for America" and "The American Family Association." I'm a member of both groups and occasionally I'll send donations to help them out. I also like to watch the "700 Club" on TV and listen to my favorite radio programs. When I hear something I don't agree with, I write or call to voice an opinion. I also send in for some of the tapes and books the guests offer because I like to keep informed.

When I was ill, I feared I would lose friends because of my sickness. For the most part it didn't happen, because when I got better I tried to explain that my odd behavior was beyond my control. But I don't think they really understood, because none of my friends experienced what I was going through when they went into menopause. So we don't talk about it much. I've noticed that it's women who are experiencing estrogen deficiency problems (either personally or because a member of their family is ill) who want to discuss it.

Our social life has changed since I got better. But that's because we spend so much time with our family. Since our friends, too, are involved with their families, it doesn't leave much time for us to get together. We've all reached a different stage of life.

Every day I thank God for leading me to Pat Simmons. She's shared a lot of her time to help me learn about diet and nutrition. By following her advice, I've been able to stop taking medicine for allergies and asthma. I'm convinced that this has improved my overall health.

I also thank God for bringing me to Dr. Tammy Geurkink, who also has become a friend. I'll never forget the day when I sat alone in the examining room waiting to see "my new doctor" and listening to footsteps walking past the room. Then I heard the chart lifted and Dr. Geurkink opened the door. She looked so beautiful and had genuine concern and compassion on her face as she looked at me. I instantly knew that I could trust her and I've never been disappointed. She took me into her care at a time when I did not know where to turn. She saw my desperation and sympathetically took time to talk to me and listen. I thank God for leading me to her.

I thank God for my writer, Judy Tremore, who has done such an excellent job in getting my book together. Without her, it would not have happened.

I also thank Him for my wonderful husband. Bob patiently struggled with me through all those horrible days and nights and never once complained about anything. He's been my friend and trusted, loving companion for almost thirty-eight years now. No woman could ask for a better husband.

And I thank You, my Heavenly Father, the Great Physician. Through Your love, You miraculously relieved me. Now I will serve You.

13

What Others Have to Say

Dear Arlene,

I'm writing this letter to you as I cry uncontrollably. I read the article in *Prevention* on "The Missing Hormone." As I read it to my husband, he said all that needed to be done was to change the name from Arlene to Carol.

For over a year and a-half now I have been in and out of hospitals. I'm presently seeing five different specialists and they all say there is nothing wrong with me—that I'm perfectly healthy and should see a psychiatrist. I'm just depressed. I'm not! It's to the point that I, too, am having daily panic attacks; it's to the point that I hate to go to bed at night because I'm afraid I'm going to die.

I'm 40 years old and had a hysterectomy three years ago. I was not given any hormones at the time.

I was glad to read your article in the magazine, because it has now given me hope. I have made an appointment with my gynecologist and hope he will read your article and give estrogen a chance with me. I was at the point where I thought there was no hope. But now,because of you, there is.

If you have any information you could give me to help me through this, or let me know what helped you get through the dizziness, panic attacks, nausea, not being able to eat, etc., please let me know.

I'm sorry this letter is so sloppy, but I'm so upset, I can't handle this much longer.

Please help with information if you can. I would love to talk to you by phone if you would call me collect.

Thank you for listening to me and helping to guide me in a new direction.

Carol
Indianapolis, Indiana

March 1991

Dear Arlene,

I am not too good at writing letters, but I must tell you. Some American friends of mine sent me your article out of the *Prevention* magazine. I can't begin to tell you how it has helped me. When I read it I thought you had written about me, with the exception that I did not have a hysterectomy. However, I had been going through menopause for eight years with no hormonal treatment. I am now fifty-four and up until the day I took ill, all I was getting was hot flashes. I thought that was bad enough, but no doctor had warned me that there were other symptoms.

I spent two weeks in two different hospitals and all they were checking was my heart (because of the rapid pounding heart beats) and also they found I have a left Bundle Block. So they didn't worry about anything else. One Sister thought I was having anxiety attacks, but no one followed that any further.

My husband took me to one of my daughter's homes 800 km (496 miles) away so I could get better medical treatment, which I did. He took blood tests and found that my estrogen level was almost nil. An ultrasound showed that my ovaries were possibly shriveled up. The doctor put me on hormone treatment and sent me to a specialist who put me on a proper course. I stayed there six weeks and then moved to another daughter's home for four weeks while sorting out the purchase of a house.

I found an excellent, caring doctor here and she has been monitoring my estrogen and updating the dosage and I am now on the mend. I still have the occasional turn, but not anywhere near as bad. But still I get scared and feel like I'm going to die. I can't wait for the time when it will all settle back to normal. It's been eight (years) now since I first took ill.

I had your article photocopied and gave one to each of the two doctors who have treated me. (Ifeel like sending them to all the doctors who didn't know what was wrong with me.)

Your article has helped me in as much as I don't feel I'm the only one that has gone through this. I know now that there is a light at the end of the tunnel—because you reached it. I carry your article in my purse as a crutch in case I ever need to tell a new doctor my problem. They can read the article and save me the long explanations.

So I want to thank you very much for writing your article. You probably never dreamed it would help someone over here in Australia.

Anita
Queensland, Australia

To *Prevention:*

I had always led a life of being in control, doing what I wanted, when I wanted. I loved my job, owned my own home, and adored gardening, reading, TV, my three dogs and the freedom that a single person enjoys. In short, I had it made. In one day, however, that all vanished.

I woke up one morning last June and couldn't get out of bed. It was as if a thief in the night had crept in and stolen my skeleton. I managed to roll out of bed and stand up, although my equilibrium was gone—like I was in moon gravity. I could walk only with my legs oddly wide apart.

As time went by, I felt faint all the time, which made me afraid to drive. I had a constant 99.3° to 99.8° fever and could no longer talk, think or write clearly. My hands would become numb. I'd get terrible heart palpitations, and there was great discomfort in my uterine area. My nights were restless and often sleepless. Life as I had known it came to a stop, and my personality changed so much that I believed I was possessed—even though I'd never before believed that was really possible.

I went to my doctor and to my therapist. Both mentioned menopause. But, at forty-six, I figured I was too young. So I dismissed that diagnosis.

Then the tests started. Blood work—nothing. Because my mother had a cancerous tumor removed at forty-five, I took an ultrasound test. Negative. A diabetes test. Negative. Week after week I became more frightened because my symptoms were getting worse. I'd wake up drenched from fear, I believed. Next diagnosis, depression. I went on the new popular drug and it changed nothing. My last desperate attempt was to get an MRI (magnetic resonance imaging test) to see if I had a brain tumor. Negative. After three months I figured I was dying. I'd spent $2,000 trying to find out what was wrong. The tests were all negative and there was nothing left to test.

I decided to start going through my home because I would be so embarrassed if the police had to come in and remove my body from the mess. I could see the headline: "Police find forty-six-year-old dead. House looks like cyclone hit it."

I started with my piled-up magazines and there, in the August 1991 "Mailbag," I saw a letter from a woman ("Story Hits Home") who'd read your article entitled The Case of the Missing Hormone (November 1990). She described symptom after symptom and I realized that I was having them all and more. All caused by estrogen deficiency.

I called my doctor the next day, who found a highly recommended gynecologist for me. The gynecologist started me on estrogen, and in five days I was well. Every symptom, except the flashes, stopped. I felt better than I had in years.

I feel like I'm a living miracle, and I owe it all to *Prevention,* my own doggedness, and the women who wrote their stories to you. I had ignored *The Case of the Missing Hormone* because I believed I was too young for menopause.

Robin
Burbank, California

Prevention:

I'm sure you don't need another menopause story, but I find it so incredible to be feeling this good that I really need to tell you why.

I am a forty-seven-year-old woman. Around Christmas time last year I lost my appetite—rare for me around the holidays. I couldn't sleep, and when I did sleep, it was troubled. I got chills, and my hands would get cold and clammy. Once I'd get going in the morning, I would hyperventilate and get light-headed. This was accompanied by extreme nervousness so severe that I couldn't sit still for two minutes. I would pace the floor for hours and drive my family crazy. I teach life skills to the handicapped, but I couldn't work because of the nervousness and lack of concentration. This whole nightmare was exacerbated by a terrible fear that crippled me so badly that I couldn't go outside.

Then I happened to read your August "Mailbag" letter called "Story Hits Home." It hadn't occurred to me that my problem could be hormonal. I was sure I had some horrible disease. I went to see a gynecologist who put me on hormone therapy. Now I feel like I've been reborn. I'm so thankful for seeing that article!

Dawn
San Francisco

Prevention:

Your November 1990 issue is one I'll never forget. I relived my own personal nightmare as I read the story of Arlene Swaney in "The Case of the Missing Hormone." You describe how it took years of suffering with nausea, nervousness and fear before a doctor figured out that the horrible symptoms were due to an estrogen deficiency after the author, Arlene, had a hysterectomy.

Except for a few minor details, I could almost substitute my name in place of hers. Even the year 1985 is the same. But I was fifty-four years of age, lived in Mississippi, and had never had a hysterectomy.

About four years after going off birth control pills my problems began almost exactly as Arlene describes. My first symptoms were a general weakness, extreme fear and nervousness. Nights of sleeplessness were soon accompanied by the "earthquake shaking from the inside." Then began the pounding of my heart, which seemed to be trying to escape from my body. Loss of appetite soon brought on weight loss.

When I visited a doctor, his diagnosis was "the beginning of a nervous collapse." I didn't see how that could be since just a few weeks earlier I had been very happy. But I tried to accept the diagnosis and took medication for depression, and later sleeping pills. But the downward spiral continued.

At one point, a friend took me to see a gynecologist. He immediately prescribed hormone medication. The fear syndrome took over, however, and I refused to have the prescription filled because someone had told me that hormones could cause cancer. Weeks moved into months as I got worse and had to spend most of my time in bed or on a recliner.

Eventually, I was sent to a psychiatrist, who changed my medication from anti-depressant to anti-anxiety. This helped for a time, and my appetite partially returned. The psychiatrist advised me to see my medical doctor weekly, and on one of these visits my doctor suggested I start the hormone medication that my gynecologist had prescribed. Now comes the miracle! Only four days on the hormones and my nervous breakdown was cured. Thanks for sharing Arlene Swaney's experience. Now I know there are others who experience the same problem.

Annie
Anguilla, Mississippi

May 1991

Dear Arlene,

Just a little gift for you on this Mother's Day to show our appreciation for all you've done for us.

I can really tell the difference and Jane is getting there too. The vitamins do play an important part, as I have found out. How nice to be able to go into stores and do things. My daughters can't believe it's their same mom and my husband just says, "Why did you waste seventeen years of your life?" I told him that's behind me and I can't change that but am so thankful for today and the days ahead of me. I am looking forward to Mother's Day this year and will sure enjoy it with my family. I have spent several Mother's Days in the hospital.

Thank you so much for writing the article, Arlene, and most of all for sharing your experiences with us. If there were only more people like you in the world, what a nice world it would be.

Love,
Marcia
Minnesota

May, 1991

Dear Arlene,

I want to thank you so much for helping Marcia and me. You know how much it means to us. I have been having a lot of problems with it for many years. The doctors have been trying to find answers. I've been through heart care and everything was fine, except for the fluid I had around the sac of the heart. I had that removed two years ago . . . They say my heart is fine. No problems at all, my heart is normal.

I still say that the fluid could have come from the progesterone I was taking with my estrogen.

When I told my doctor, he just said stop taking it if you feel that way about it. This really got me upset with him. After my last visit with the heart doctor, he told me everything was fine and I should take nerve pills and go see a psychologist.

After all this, Marcia and I started to get together more and talk about everything, trying to find answers to all of our problems.

I know that day she got her *Prevention,* she called about your story and asked me if I got a chance to read mine yet. I said, no, so right there on the spot, I got my book and read it all. I know at first we just kept talking about it (because) we were really having a bad time. (Then one afternoon) your story in *Prevention* came up again and I said, "If it wasn't for the farm, I would go out to Michigan right now." I felt I couldn't take time off.

That night Marcia called and said, "Did you mean what you said this afternoon?"

I thought for a second and said, "Yes, what are we waiting for? We've been putting up with this for so long. Let's see if we can get some answers."

We talked of what we would do. If we could get our doctor to go along with us, we'd do it all with his support. If he wouldn't go along, we would either fly or drive out your way. So our first step was to get the doctor's opinion of your story in Prevention . . . .

Our next step was to call you. However, we didn't know if we would be able to reach you. After we had spoken with you my son said, "Mom, weren't you and Marcia scared that Arlene wasn't around anymore or maybe was even dead?" I said, "You bet! All kinds of thoughts went through our heads." The rest you know.

Our families are both a lot more at peace, knowing and understanding what's going on; it's such a great help since this has been hard on them.

Thanks again. We are on the complete program now, so time will tell. It has helped somewhat—you know how it all works . . . I get sleepy a lot and run out of power to move my body.

Have a Happy Mother's Day. Sure wish there were more people like you around. Would make this whole world a lot happier.

Love,
Jane
Minnesota

December 1991

Dear Arlene,

Thanks again for your help. I've been feeling one-hundred percent better and can handle stress better. Saturday I went shopping . . . and it was so warm . . . I had my coat off, but got so warm it turned my stomach so we headed home. Haven't had one like that for a long time so I didn't complain.

. . . A lady down my street is also on the program. She came over last night to talk to me. She needed some reassurance that she isn't the only one and "no, it is not in your head." She's going to our doctor on Thursday and felt better when she left my house. We are so thankful for your article. You have touched many lives.

Marcia
Minnesota

November 1992

Dear Arlene,

It's been very hectic for Jane and me this past summer and fall. Had some rough days. No, we are no longer on the patch. Our doctor left our clinic . . . . What an adjustment for us. Our new doctor spent time on the phone with Dr. Tammy who told her to ask the other doctor to give us depo-Estradiol and not the patch. We have increased the depo-Estradiol because the shot wasn't lasting long enough. We get them every two-to-three weeks and hopefully can go four-to-six weeks once our bodies catch up. Dr. Tammy has several women who come once a week for this shot. She said stress drains the estrogen very fast. My mom had surgery on October 6 . . . She needed 24-hour care and I'm the only child, so you can see where my estrogen went fast . . . .

Jane arranged with a college for us to do seminars on menopause. Not too many women are willing to talk about their problems. But we are more than willing to share ours—what we have gone through since all this started and how we found help . . . .

Jane's counselor talked to us several times and thought we should do this. She has many clients who have lots of questions. We have all the books and pamphlets that we bought or ordered, even tapes that help to relax you. We're very anxious to get started. Jane and I decided that we would demand a well-ventilated room since neither of us can stand closed in places.

Love,
Marcia
Minnesota

May 1991

Dear Arlene,

Thank you for taking the time to talk to me and send me literature. Thank you so much for writing that article in *Prevention* and giving me Marcia's phone number. I have been in touch with her also. I feel better just knowing you and Marcia are there for support.

I have not had luck finding a doctor but I do have a GYN appointment with a doctor recommended by the North American Menopause Society of America. I couldn't believe it when I saw one doctor in my clinic and hope to heaven he will listen to me.

I hope you are doing well. I am going out looking at vitamins today. I wish I knew what vitamins you are taking. Do you take a B complex or a stress combination?

I feel very anxious a lot of the time and jump inside, but I do feel somewhat better after two months on the patch. I'm having off-balance feelings and, or "an episode" as I call my feelings now, about once a week and not as bad. But I don't want *any*. I wonder if I'll ever feel good again.

Darlene
Minneapolis

February 1992

Dear Arlene,

I'll bet you're surprised to hear from me so soon. I had to call and tell you that right after I sent your last letter, I had a very bad episode on Valentine's Day afternoon to be exact. What happened was I got on my mini-tramp and stayed on it through a half-hour show. I came upstairs, sat down and whammo, I got so dizzy and nauseated, with flutters across my chest, and my arms and fingers started tingling. I was so unprepared for this after almost a year. I was scared to death. All that jumping up and down must have brought it on.

I called Marcia and talked to her for half an hour for support. She said two weeks ago she crawled on her hands and knees to the kitchen to turn off her stove. I told her it was not very encouraging after eighteen years wearing the patch and being on estrogen shots. She's still having problems, but she says she is a lot better, and so am. It's been almost a year, so I'm grateful for that.

I wish there were support groups for this problem. I was thinking of writing to *Prevention*. They have a lot of feedback from your article and maybe that way we could find each other. I feel so alone with this; I wish you lived next to me and

Marcia and Jane so we could talk and support each other often, but we're only a phone call and letter away. No one really understands unless they have the problem. Thanks again for writing that article.

Darlene
Minneapolis

P.S. It's Monday the 17th and I have a fuzzy band around my head, but otherwise I've had a good day at work. I started at 9:30 and it's now 4:30, so it's not bad like it was one year ago. Thank you God.

Other Books by Starburst Publishers

(Partial listing—full list available on request)

Health, Happiness & Hormones —Arlene Swaney

Subtitled: *One Woman's Journey Toward Health After a Hysterectomy.* A frightening and candid look into one woman's struggle to find a cure for her medical condition. In 1990, when her story was first published in *Prevention* magazine, author Arlene Swaney received an overwhelming response from women who also were plagued by mysterious, but familiar, symptoms leading to continuous misdiagnoses. Starting with a hysterectomy Swaney details the years of lost health that followed as she searched for an accurate diagnosis. Her story is told with warmth and compassion.

(trade paper) ISBN 0914984721 **$9.95**

Migraine—Winning The Fight of Your Life —Charles Theisler

This book describes the hurt, loneliness and agony that migraine sufferers experience and the difficulty they must live with. It explains the different types of migraines and their symptoms, as well as the related health hazards. Gives 200 ways to help fight off migraines, and shows how to experience fewer headaches, reduce their duration, and decrease the agony and pain involved.

(trade paper) ISBN 0914984632 **$10.95**

The World's Oldest Health Plan —Kathleen O'Bannon Baldinger

Subtitled: *Health, Nutrition and Healing from the Bible.* Offers a complete health plan for body, mind and spirit, just as Jesus did. It includes programs for diet, exercise and mental health. Contains foods and recipes to lower cholesterol and blood pressure, improve the immune system and other bodily functions, reduce stress, reduce or cure constipation, eliminate insomnia, reduce forgetfulness, confusion and anger, increase circulation and thinking ability, eliminate "yeast" problems, improve digestion, and much more.

(trade paper-opens flat) ISBN 0914984578 **$14.95**

Dr. Kaplan's Lifestyle of the Fit & Famous —Eric Scott Kaplan

Subtitled: *A Wellness Approach to "Thinning and Winning."* A comprehensive guide to the formulas and principles of: FAT LOSS, EXERCISE, VITAMINS, NATURAL HEALTH, SUCCESS and HAPPINESS. More than a health book—it is a lifestyle based on the empirical formulas of healthy living. Dr. Kaplan's food-combining principles take into account all the major food sources (fats, proteins, carbohydrates, sugars, etc.) that when combined within the proper formula (e.g. proteins cannot be mixed with refined carbohydrates) will increase metabolism and decrease the waistline. This allows you to eat the foods you want, feel great, and eliminate craving and binging.

(hard cover) ISBN 091498456X **$21.95**

Books by Starburst Publishers—cont'd.

Allergy Cooking With Ease —Nicolette M. Dumke

Subtitled: *The No Wheat, Milk, Eggs, Corn, Soy, Yeast, Sugar, Grain, and Gluten Cookbook.* A book designed to provide a wide variety of recipes to meet many different types of dietary and social needs and, whenever possible, save you time in food preparation. Includes: Recipes for those special foods that most food allergy patients think they will never eat again; Timesaving tricks; and Allergen Avoidance Index.

(trade paper-opens flat) ISBN 091498442X **$12.95**

God's Vitamin "C" for the Spirit

—Kathy Collard Miller & D. Larry Miller

Subtitled: *"Tug-at-the-Heart" Stories to Fortify and Enrich Your Life.* Includes inspiring stories and anecdotes that emphasize Christian ideals and values by Barbara Johnson, Billy Graham, Nancy L. Dorner, Dave Dravecky, Patsy Clairmont, Charles Swindoll, H. Norman Wright, Adell Harvey, Max Lucado, James Dobson, Jack Hayford and many other well-known Christian speakers and writers. Topics include: Love, Family Life, Faith and Trust, Prayer, Marriage, Relationships, Grief, Spiritual Life, Perseverance, Christian Living, and God's Guidance.

(trade paper) ISBN 0914984837 **$12.95**

God's Chewable Vitamin "C" for the Spirit

Subtitled: *A Dose of God's Wisdom One Bite at a Time.* A collection of inspirational Quotes and Scriptures by many of your favorite Christian speakers and writers. It will motivate your life and inspire your spirit. You will *chew* on every bite of **God's Chewable Vitamin "C" for the Spirit.**

(trade paper) ISBN 0914984845 **$6.95**

Purchasing Information:

Books are available from your favorite Bookstore, either from current stock or special order. To assist bookstore in locating your selection be sure to give title, author, and ISBN #. If unable to purchase from the bookstore you may order direct from STARBURST PUBLISHERS. When ordering enclose full payment plus $3.00 for shipping and handling ($4.00 if Canada or Overseas). Payment in US Funds only. Please allow two to three weeks minimum (longer overseas) for delivery. Make checks payable to and mail to STARBURST PUBLISHERS, P.O. Box 4123, LANCASTER, PA 17604. Credit card orders may also be placed by calling 1-800-441-1456 (credit card orders only), Mon-Fri, 8 AM–5 PM Eastern Time. **Prices and availability subject to change without notice.** 1-96